THE
LITTLE BOOK
OF
CANNABIS

HOW MARIJUANA CAN
IMPROVE YOUR LIFE

· · · · · ·

AMANDA SIEBERT
FOREWORD BY **DR. RAV IVKER**

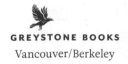

GREYSTONE BOOKS
Vancouver/Berkeley

To the patients who are suffering, the enthusiasts standing up to adversity, the activists decrying unjust laws, and those doing time for victimless crimes: this book is for you.

· · · · · ·

Greystone Books Ltd.
greystonebooks.com

Cataloguing data available from Library and Archives Canada
ISBN 978-1-77164-404-4 (pbk.)
ISBN 978-1-77164-405-1 (epub)

Editing by Eva van Emden
Cover design and illustrations by Brian Tong
Text design by Nayeli Jimenez
Printed and bound in Canada on ancient-forest-friendly paper by Friesens

Greystone Books gratefully acknowledges the Musqueam, Squamish, and Tsleil-Waututh peoples on whose land our office is located.

Greystone Books thanks the Canada Council for the Arts, the British Columbia Arts Council, the Province of British Columbia through the Book Publishing Tax Credit, and the Government of Canada for supporting our publishing activities.

Canadä

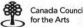

For more information including tips and how-to's, visit littlebookofcannabis.com.

CONTENTS

...

DISCLAIMER

...

THIS BOOK IS not intended to be a substitute for medical advice from physicians. The reader should regularly consult a physician about matters relating to their health, and particularly with respect to any symptoms that may require diagnosis or medical attention. While this book may mention specific product types, cannabis strains, cannabinoids, consumption methods, and so forth, the author and publisher recommend that readers notify their physicians if they are thinking about consuming cannabis for medicinal purposes.

Although the author and publisher have made every effort to ensure that the information in this book was correct at press time, they do not assume, and hereby disclaim, any liability to any part for any loss, damage, or disruption caused by errors or omissions, whether such errors or omissions result from negligence, accident, or any other cause.

The state of cannabis research is changing, and with the renewed interest in this plant, it is being studied more rigorously. As such, future research on the topics mentioned may come to conclusions that are contrary to what has been printed in this book.

Please consult local laws for the minimum age for cannabis use and other restrictions.

...

FOREWORD

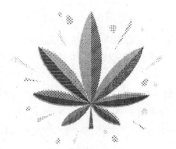

THIS HIGHLY INFORMATIVE book provides readers, first-timers as well as experienced consumers, with an excellent practical introduction to the multifaceted life-changing benefits of cannabis.

Retail sales of cannabis began in Canada on October 17, 2018, making it the second nation in the world, after Uruguay, to legalize the herb for recreational use. Since 2001, medical marijuana has been legal in Canada, as it is in the majority of U.S. states, at time of writing, with an ever-increasing number also approving the use of recreational cannabis. This rapidly accelerating trend is reversing nearly a century of prohibition of a powerful medicinal herb used throughout the world both medically and spiritually for more than five thousand years.

However, as a result of its illegality, its criminalization, and the lack of knowledge about the circumstances that led to its prohibition, as well as disapproval among the medical establishment, the majority of the world's current population under-standably remains skeptical. In addition, there has been a relative lack of reliable evidence-based information to dispel the myths and misconceptions surrounding cannabis. *The Little Book of Cannabis* helps significantly to fill that void.

As a holistic physician and cannabis clinician, I have used medical marijuana with more than eight thousand patients to relieve their suffering. From both my professional and personal experience with cannabis, spanning more than five decades, I strongly support the material presented by Amanda Siebert. Whether the chapter is discussing the use of cannabis for insomnia, anxiety, pain, inflammation, cancer, creativity and sexual pleasure, or end-of-life care, the author offers valuable and accurate information. I enjoyed her real-life compelling case studies, which correlated well with many of my patient stories.

By far the most frequent use of cannabis as a medicine, and its greatest therapeutic benefit, is the relief of chronic pain. This is certainly true of my practice, as more than 90 percent of my patients suffer with some degree of persistent pain. I found Chapter 7, "An Effective Source of Pain Management," to be particularly helpful for any patient struggling with chronic pain or physicians who might be hesitant about treating their patients with cannabis. Siebert did a superb job of researching this topic, drawing heavily on recent studies, historical references, and the work of Dr. Mark Ware, an associate professor in family medicine and anesthesia at McGill University in Montreal and the director of clinical research at the Alan Edwards Pain Management Unit at the McGill University Health Centre.

As a physician, I found the scientific references to be of particular interest, and they added to my knowledge base. The book is very well written, well researched, concise, yet comprehensive in its scope of cannabis-related quality-of-life benefits. Cannabis is a complex herb containing more than two hundred compounds. Siebert is able to simplify its complexity and provide explanations at a level that can be easily understood by most readers. As a result, *The Little Book of Cannabis* is an excellent guide for anyone interested in using this remarkable herb to heighten their enjoyment of life.

DR. RAV IVKER
Author, *Cannabis for Chronic Pain*
Cofounder and former president, American Board of Integrative Holistic Medicine

. . .

INTRODUCTION

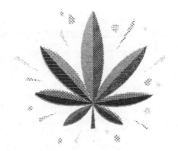

WHILE MY AGE of introduction to cannabis might send a shudder down the spine of any lawmaker considering the pros and cons of cannabis legalization, the stigma associated with youth use is one of the reasons I feel the need to share my experience. At age fourteen, while taking a break from staffing the merch table at a local punk show in my hometown of Richmond, B.C., I tried cannabis for the first time. I had been curious about the strange weed that my parents had cautioned me to avoid, but when my older friends said it helped them feel relaxed, I figured my parents were wrong and, like so many teenagers do, I decided I had to find out for myself if cannabis would indeed "fry my brain cells." Seated atop a picnic table with two girlfriends, I indulged in a hoot and a half from a pipe, which resulted in a momentary fit of laughter but nothing more. After that first encounter, I used cannabis occasionally in social settings with friends, but it wasn't until college that I began to discover how using it brought me direct and indirect benefits in other areas of my life.

I remember walking into a friend's house for the first time during my second year of college and seeing him point to a set of roach clips on the table. (For the uninitiated, these are used to hold a joint when it gets too short to smoke holding it with your fingers.) I remember thinking, "Wow, this weed stuff can get pretty hardcore." I won't lie; there was a little judgment there—and then I got high. From that point on, everything changed.

It wasn't long before I began to appreciate cannabis for its ability to stoke conversation at social gatherings and calm me down after a week of late nights spent meeting tight deadlines. Friday and Saturday evenings were often spent steeped in bubbles of intelligent thought and clouds of cannabis smoke as my friends and I waxed poetic about our studies, current events, and pop culture, often opting for doobies over booze in the interest of avoiding the next day's hangover. Soon, when assignments started to pile up, part-time shifts at work gobbled up my free time, and arguments with my mother (sorry, Mom) took me to the edge, cannabis would bring me to a place where all the seemingly impossible tasks of the day could be tackled with a puff and a simple shift in perspective.

I would soon discover that, even in the depths of a spinning anxiety attack or a lapse in judgment caused by a stress-induced outburst, the plant my parents, teachers, and authorities were so vehemently opposed to was able to bring me more than just relaxation—it brought me peace of mind.

Then, while writing this book, I was diagnosed with PTSD (post-traumatic stress disorder), generalized anxiety disorder, and depression. The symptoms of my conditions nearly put me over the edge, but I told myself I could manage and that I didn't have time in my busy schedule to find help. I chose to wear my struggle on the inside until I interviewed Dr. Zach Walsh on the subject of PTSD while experiencing the very symptoms he listed off. That's when I realized that it was time I put my health first. (Thankfully, my editors and publishers were incredibly understanding of this situation.) Everything changed again, but in a much different way as I began using cannabis with a new intention: relieving the flashbacks, panic attacks, and "hair trigger" you'll read about in Chapter 3. And while cannabis has certainly been there to help lift my mood, relieve my anxiety, and calm my erratic nerves, I used it frequently in the process of writing this book to help spur creative thought, too.

Having said all of this, writing a book about cannabis was never something I seriously considered until it fell into my lap. While my day job at a newspaper had me neck-deep in cannabis policy announcements, news of corporate mergers, and the unending flow of information on Twitter, writing this book allowed me to gain a deeper understanding of exactly what cannabis does when it enters the body, and how we as humans can use its healing properties to treat different ailments, relieve stress, and even spice up our sex lives. (Trust me on this one. Skip to Chapter 6 if you must.) My appreciation for the plant that has brought so much improvement to my life has grown, you might say, like the very weed in question.

But every time I get excited about cannabis and its potential, I'm reminded that it's only truly accessible in a few areas of the world. The global war on drugs, and on cannabis in particular, has resulted in the arrest of hundreds of thousands of people. More than half of drug arrests in the United States are related to cannabis. Between 2001 and 2010, 8.2 million Americans were arrested for cannabis-related offences, with 88 percent of those being for simple possession. These arrests cause irreparable harm to families and communities and occur at disproportionate rates among people of color.[1] The same is true in Canada,[2] where in 2016—the year after Prime Minister Justin Trudeau promised to legalize cannabis—55,000 cannabis-related charges were laid, with 76 percent for simple possession.[3] That a plant—put here by God, you might

THE LITTLE BOOK OF CANNABIS

say—with such incredible medical benefits has been vilified truly upsets me, and that people continue to be unjustifiably punished for using it angers me to my core.

My personal experience with the plant is just one perspective, but when it's combined with the testimony of the hundreds of people I've met, interviewed, and smoked with, as well as the bodies of research that scientists have been trying to develop for the last several decades, the benefits of using it become too great to ignore—as do the grave and inherent harms associated with its prohibition. When we add the historical uses of cannabis to all of our current evidence, the idea that this plant is illegal *anywhere* in the world becomes preposterous. In truth, the last seventy-five to one hundred years are the aberration. Cannabis is only the forbidden herb we know it to be because in the 1930s, a few powerful men crafted some artful propaganda, and it became accepted as fact. Historically, cannabis was used to treat a variety of illnesses dating back thousands of years, and as recently as the mid-1800s it was a mainstay in medicine cabinets throughout North America.

It is my hope that those who read this book approach this material with an open mind, and perhaps with a willingness to shed the negative messages they've carried about cannabis from the past. For years, we've been fed misinformation about a plant that in many cases is nothing short of life-saving. I hope that this little act of rebellion (after all, this *is* a book about a controversial substance) opens your mind to the idea that cannabis is more than just a weed with an undeserved reputation—it's a plant that truly does hold the power to improve your life.

1
...

IMPROVING SLEEP

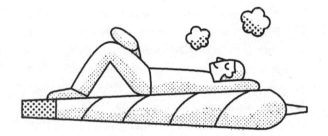

Case Study: Guilherme Falcão

....

FOR AS LONG as Guilherme Falcão can remember (that is, as early as age seven), he's had trouble falling asleep at night.

"Since I was a kid, I've had a problem staying focused and issues with anxiety," the twenty-nine-year-old tells me. Add a young brain that just doesn't seem to have an off-switch and you have the perfect recipe for countless sleepless nights spent lying awake, staring at the ceiling. Time and place didn't seem to make a difference, and even if Falcão was in bed with his head on the pillow by 10 p.m., sleep would often evade him until two or three in the morning.

Struggling with insomnia as an adult is one thing, but when I ask him about the effects that insomnia had on his childhood, his voice lowers, and I can sense his feelings of frustration.

"I was *always* tired as a kid," he says. "I never wanted to get up and go to school, because I'd only ever get two or three hours of sleep." And even when sleep did come, what little shut-eye he did get was of rather poor quality.

It wasn't until Falcão was a young adult that a doctor recommended he try using sleeping pills.

"The medication made it easy to get to sleep," he says, "but it was very, very hard to wake up. Every day, I felt horrible side effects—I was always tired, dizzy, or nauseous—it's why I didn't take them every night; just when I really, really couldn't fall asleep."

One night in his early twenties, while out with a friend, Falcão had his first taste of cannabis. He enjoyed the wave of relaxation he felt wash over him, but had no idea of the plant's potential therapeutic effects. He went home to bed, and what happened next came as a complete surprise.

"That night, I had one of the best sleeps of my whole life," he says. "I've been using weed to help me fall asleep ever since."

Since making the switch from sleeping pills to cannabis, he says he's yet to experience a negative side effect—save for an adjustment to his tolerance to cannabis, an effect any regular cannabis user, and in fact many regular users of pharmaceutical drugs, encounter.

These days, he says he gets an average of five to seven hours of uninterrupted sleep a night, a quantum leap in quality and quantity compared to the two or three measly hours a night he'd get as a child. Falcão says the positive effects of quality sleep every night have trickled into every aspect of his life.

"I have way more energy because I'm sleeping much better. I think I'm happier now too, because I can have a whole night of sleep, I can focus in the morning, and I can do my work effectively—things that I couldn't do before, because I was always tired or under the effects of sleeping pills."

Why So Sleep Deprived?

WHEN WE'RE STANDING in line in the grocery store, health magazines promoting self-improvement in areas like diet, exercise, and productivity regularly get our attention, but it seems to me that sleep isn't often part of the conversation. Make no mistake: poor sleep is the big elephant in the room when it comes to what's causing many of North America's most common diseases, including obesity, cardiovascular disease, type 2 diabetes, depression, and overall reduced well-being.

All it takes to size up North America's problem with sleep is a look at its penchant for sleep aids. The largest-ever consumer sleep study conducted in the United States revealed in 2017 that 50 percent of adults reported using a mix of two or more sleep aids per night, such as prescription medications, over-the-counter sleeping pills, or herbal remedies and food supplements. Even then, 79 percent of respondents said they got less sleep than the recommended seven hours per night.[1] In Canada, the problem is less severe, with about one-third of the population sleeping for fewer than the recommended number of hours, but in a representative survey of the population, almost 50 percent said they have issues falling asleep or staying asleep.[2]

Given the consequences of poor or insufficient sleep, this reliance on sleep aids makes sense. We know that eventually, lack of quality sleep can catch up with us and lead to disease, but lack of sleep affects us in the short term, too. How many times have you found yourself plugging away in your cubicle when a wave of brain fog stops you dead in your tracks? Unfortunately, having trouble focusing is just the tip of the iceberg: sleep deprivation also leads to mood swings, a weakened immune system, high blood pressure, weight gain, poor balance, and low libido.

Even when we *think* we're getting enough sleep, environmental factors like light, sound, and stress can affect the quality of that sleep, reducing the value of the hours we spend in bed and possibly leaving us feeling groggier than before. Few things are more frustrating than making the time to hit the sheets early only to find yourself lying awake contemplating the state of the world until three in the morning. Or you might fall asleep quickly but find you wake up intermittently, perhaps because of a snoring partner or nagging pain. Whatever is keeping you from getting a good night's rest, interrupted sleep can be profoundly exasperating and can leave you feeling powerless and fatigued.

Experiencing a rough night's sleep every now and then is common, but some people are affected by sleep disorders that can wreak havoc on their day-to-day lives. Insomnia, sleep apnea, restless leg syndrome, and narcolepsy are just a few common sleep disorders that can be caused by a combination of factors ranging from physical and medical issues to psychiatric disorders and environmental factors. They also come with brutal side effects that can include depression, anxiety, fatigue, lowered immunity, hormonal disruption, and hallucinations. While pharmaceuticals can offer relief for some of these conditions, they often come with their own disruptive side effects.

Poor sleep has the potential to completely derail a healthy lifestyle, so correcting a faulty sleep pattern is the best way to improve overall health and well-being. In my discussions with physicians, many have explained that one of the first symptoms they look to treat, regardless of the condition or disorder in question, is their patients' fatigue and exhaustion. They tell me it's the most important step in restoring their patients to optimum levels of health, because when the body has the opportunity to rest properly, it can heal more effectively and more efficiently.

To correct our poor sleep problems, it's important to know where the problems might be coming from, and in order to do that, we must first understand the different stages of sleep. The first stage begins once you've made the decision to go to sleep and you've closed your eyes. During this short period, you may drift into sleep, but you're able to return to a state of wakefulness if necessary. During the subsequent stage, your heart rate and metabolic processes slow down and your body temperature begins to decrease. A person with severe sleep deprivation might skip past these stages straight to stage three, what sleep specialists refer to as "slow-wave sleep." At this stage, it becomes more challenging for external stimuli to disrupt a person's sleep. This is the stage at which the brain releases growth hormones that stimulate tissue growth and muscle repair. According to a Harvard Medical School report on improving sleep, young people spend about 20 percent of their sleep time in this stage, but for most people, by age sixty five, it becomes "nearly absent."[3] The final stage, REM or "rapid eye movement" sleep, is the stage when vivid dreams occur. These are usually the dreams we remember the next day. Typically, slow-wave and REM sleep are considered the most important for maintaining good physical and mental health.

Interruptions to your sleep cycle might leave you feeling desperate for solutions, and while sleeping pills might be helpful in the short term, they can be addictive and commonly cause side effects like constipation, changes in appetite, dry mouth, unwanted drowsiness, heartburn, stomach pains, and physical weakness; repeated use can even lead to memory loss. One study from 2012 estimated that sleeping pills were associated with as many as 507,000 deaths in the U.S. that year.[4] By comparing the death rates among people who had taken sleeping pills and people who had not, the study found that even when patients were prescribed as few as eighteen sleeping pills per year, medications like zolpidem could increase their likelihood of death by as much as three times. Given the importance of sleep, however, the side effects of sleeping pills don't seem to deter people from taking them and doctors from prescribing them: between 2006 and 2011, the number of sleeping pill prescriptions in the United States rose from forty-seven million to sixty million.

Historical Use of Cannabis for Sleep

CANNABIS HAD MANY uses in ancient India, and traditional Ayurvedic medicinal texts written during the eleventh century maintained that it had strong soporific, or sleep-inducing, qualities. While insomniacs of today might prefer to smoke or vaporize a high-THC strain to fall asleep faster, consumption methods in 600 BCE weren't quite the same. At that time, cannabis was likely smoked over a large fire in groups (imagine a session in which giant bales of cannabis were burned while people inhaled the resulting smoke) or prepared and served in a ritual drink made with *bhang*, a paste made from cannabis buds and leaves. By the time the Indian Hemp Drugs Commission heard testimony in 1893 that cannabis could be used as a sedative and to counteract insomnia, tinctures of cannabis were being used widely by doctors thanks to William O'Shaughnessy.

The first official use of a cannabis tincture took place in 1843, when the Irish doctor published a study based on his experience with the preparation and included a recipe for others to use.[5] It wasn't long before physicians considered its use for their sleep-deprived patients. In 1860, Dr. R.R. M'Meens reviewed the literature of the time and reported it to the Ohio State Medical Society, writing that in some cases, the less intense side effects of cannabis made it his preferred choice over opium: "The whole effect of hemp being less violent, and producing a more natural sleep, without interfering with the actions of the internal organs, it is certainly often preferable to opium, although it is not equal to that drug in strength and reliability," he wrote.[6] As such, cannabis tinctures were often prescribed for insomnia and other sleep-related issues. Even Sir J. Russell Reynolds, Queen Victoria's physician, administered cannabis as a sedative and said that very small doses were often all that were required. In four pages of the 1868 *U.S. Dispensatory* dedicated to *extractum cannabis*, the authors lauded the plant for its ability to induce sleep.

While past research largely centers on sleep as a whole, up-to-date research takes a more nuanced approach by considering the effects of cannabis on the various stages of sleep, and whether those effects might disrupt other areas of the mind and body. It might be a widely held belief among cannabis users that a quick puff before bed can facilitate falling asleep, and even help someone stay asleep, but among researchers, opinions on the relationship between sleep and cannabis vary.

How Cannabis Can Help

WHILE THERE'S NO arguing with the fact that cannabis affects sleep, researchers are still working to determine which stages of sleep are affected by cannabis, and which combination of compounds of the plant are most likely to help someone achieve a long, satisfying night of rest. These are cannabinoids, the potent molecules in cannabis that give it its medicinal value. The most commonly investigated cannabinoids are THC (tetrahydrocannabinol) and CBD (cannabidiol), and both have been shown to have applications as sleep aids.

Before we explore how these cannabinoids can affect sleep, let's consider how many people find cannabis to be an effective sleep aid. In a 2016 survey of patients conducted by HelloMD, an online platform for medical cannabis users, insomnia was among the top three most common conditions being treated, with 65 percent of respondents saying they used cannabis to help them fall asleep. Patients who used cannabis for other conditions listed better sleep as a common beneficial side effect, with 79 percent of respondents agreeing that it helped them sleep better.[7] In a Canadian study of 628 people who used cannabis for therapeutic purposes, 85 percent said they used cannabis to address issues with sleep, as well as other problems like pain and anxiety.[8] Pain is often the most cited reason for using cannabis, and it frequently goes together with sleep problems. Pain can interrupt sleep and lead to a lack of slow-wave and REM sleep, causing more problems for the patient overall. Pain sufferers often report that when they started using cannabis, both their pain and their sleep schedules improved.

There are a few things we can say for sure about

cannabis and sleep. One of cannabis's most popular cannabinoids, THC, has been shown to dramatically increase melatonin production in the brain, a naturally occurring hormone that regulates the body's circadian rhythm.[9] (If you've ever struggled with jetlag, a doctor might have recommended melatonin supplements to help get your sleep schedule back on track.) When cannabinoids like THC and CBD enter the body, they mimic compounds that the body makes, called endocannabinoids. These neurochemicals are a critical aspect of the body's endocannabinoid system, which is responsible for a host of bodily functions, including the regulation of sleep. (For more info on the endocannabinoid system, check out Appendix 1.) When it comes to inducing sleep, a 1973 study of otherwise healthy insomniacs published in the journal *Psychopharmacologia* showed that THC could decrease the time it takes to fall asleep—sleep latency—by over one hour. Researchers also associated doses of THC with a decrease in sleep interruptions during the first half of the night.[10]

Since then, the efficacy of cannabis, and specifically THC, in initiating sleep has been reiterated in several studies. An article in 2017 noted that THC could "reduce sleep onset latency in naïve users or at low doses in experienced users," but that high doses in experienced users could actually increase sleep latency.[11]

Another study that found that the use of smoked cannabis or oral THC helped subjects fall asleep also found that it lengthened the amount of time subjects spent in slow-wave sleep and reduced the time spent in REM sleep.[12] This is where the science on cannabis and sleep can get a little complicated.

At HelloMD, Dr. Perry Solomon encounters a lot of questions about cannabis and sleep. He says that while some physicians emphasize the importance of the REM stage, the benefits of more time in slow-wave sleep shouldn't be overlooked, especially in older patients who might already be losing out on this kind of sleep.

"Slow-wave sleep is thought to be the most restorative, and cannabis can lengthen that restoration phase," he says of the stage thought to be most sensitive to the influence of cannabis. "In theory, it can reduce the plaque and the beta-amyloids in the... brain, which can lead to Alzheimer's disease."

So should cannabis users worry if they're simply trading one form of deep sleep for another? After all, the purpose of REM sleep is still up for debate—some subscribe to the idea that REM sleep regulates neurotransmitters and body temperature, while others think it helps the brain form new memories. Although less REM sleep might mean less dreaming, researchers still aren't sure whether disruptions to REM sleep lead to issues for users.[13]

Traditionally, THC-dominant products were thought to be helpful for inducing sleep, but scientists have now learned that CBD might have value in this arena as well, though some results are contradictory. CBD, a nonintoxicating compound in cannabis, has significant medical benefits and can actually counter the "high" that users feel when they consume THC. One of the earliest reviews of the efficacy of CBD looked at its use among healthy volunteers, insomniacs, and epileptic patients, and found it has properties as a sedative, anticonvulsant, and anti-inflammatory.[14] This finding has been backed up in several subsequent studies, which also found that while CBD counters the euphoria caused by THC, it potentiates the sedative effects of THC, making them stronger.

Before we dissect CBD and its effects on sleep, let's take a second to look at the interactions between THC and CBD. Scientists theorize that these and dozens of other cannabinoids in cannabis have complementary effects on each other, creating an interactive synergy referred to as the entourage effect. This synergy implies that the best cannabis medicine is one that uses all parts of the plant. In short, it's a classic case of the whole—that is, cannabis—being greater than the sum of its parts—that is, THC and CBD.

If we look at more recent studies that have examined the efficacy of CBD on a surface level, we

might actually conclude that it promotes wakefulness. But a deep dive into the data reveals that the
effects of CBD are biphasic, meaning that at low
doses CBD acts as a stimulant, and at higher doses
it acts as a sedative. For example, when subjects
in a 2004 study were given low doses of CBD—just
15 milligrams per day before bed—it made them
more alert.[15] But in the study we mentioned earlier, where subjects were given doses of CBD of
40, 80, and 160 milligrams per day, sleep time
was increased and sleep interruptions were less
frequent.[16]

The science around cannabis and sleep disorders is a little more nuanced. Given THC's ability to
help people fall asleep faster, researchers agree that
it has potential for people suffering from insomnia. And while nightmares in patients with PTSD
are not technically a sleep disorder, studies have
shown that synthetic THC can significantly reduce
these nightmares.[17] Patients with sleep apnea could
also potentially find relief with THC.[18] Narcolepsy,
on the other hand, might be best treated using the
cannabinoid CBD because of its ability to induce
wakefulness.[19]

Using Cannabis for Sleep

BEYOND OUR KNOWLEDGE of the effects of THC
and CBD on sleep, there are a few ideas about which

types of cannabis work best that cannabis users often debate, but before we get into specifics, consider your sleep pattern and try to decide what needs to be changed: Are you having problems falling asleep, or staying asleep? The answer to this question will determine your best course of action.

Let's say, you're having a hard time falling asleep, and you're interested in giving smoked or vaporized cannabis a shot. A budtender at a dispensary will almost always suggest that cannabis categorized as indica rather than sativa will serve as a better sleep aid, but as we begin to understand how other compounds within the plant affect us, these classifications are secondary to the cannabinoid and terpene profiles, which list the amount of various cannabinoids and terpenes (the aromatic compounds in cannabis that give it its distinct smell) within a certain strain or medicine. If you want to know exactly which ones are in your cannabis, ask the budtender for the cannabinoid and terpene profiles. A good dispensary will be transparent with its members. Three popular nighttime strains are God's Gift, Northern Lights, and Death Bubba. They're all indica-dominant strains that put THC's sleep-inducing qualities front and center, and also contain myrcene, a terpene thought to induce sleep.

Given the research, we know that what might be useful for a novice cannabis user looking to fall asleep faster might not work for an established user: low doses of THC have been shown to sedate effectively, but for people with a higher tolerance, a vastly different dose might be required for the same effect. While some cannabis users swear by regular breaks from THC products to avoid building up a tolerance to the plant's dominant compound, others prefer to use a mix of THC- and CBD-dominant products.

A person with absolutely no history of cannabis use might find that CBD-dominant products that contain a very low dose of THC might present a better option—keeping in mind not only that low doses of CBD can lead to wakefulness, but also that CBD can potentiate the sedative effects of THC. A good choice might be a strain like ACDC or a tincture with a high ratio of CBD to THC.

Because the quickest way to deliver cannabinoids to the body is by smoking or vaporizing cannabis, these are considered the best consumption methods if you're looking to induce sleep. But if your problem is staying asleep rather than falling asleep, you might want to consider edible products like tinctures or capsules. (Food products are also an option, but be wary of options with a lot of sugar, which could have an adverse effect on your sleep.) It takes longer to feel the onset of effects from an edible product, but the effects last longer and can manifest differently than the euphoria caused by simply smoking or vaporizing: while smoking might make you feel a little heady, you'll feel the effects of an edible in your whole body. For this reason, a patient who is woken up nightly by chronic pain might find more relief from an edible than from a smokeable. Since cannabinoids like THC and CBD are fat-soluble, it's best to take them with a fatty snack, although having too much food in your stomach might extend the length of time it takes for you to feel the effects. At HelloMD, Solomon and his colleagues tell patients to keep a sleep journal that tracks their last meal of the day, when they go to bed, when they fall asleep, which products and cannabinoids they're using, and how long they sleep for. He recommends that they maintain their journal until they can find a dose that works consistently.

DECREASING STRESS AND ANXIETY

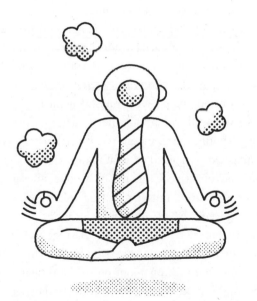

Case Study: Piper Courtenay

IT'S NOT OFTEN you meet someone willing to talk openly about their personal struggles without the fear of being stigmatized, but the first time I met Piper Courtenay, a fellow writer also thoroughly immersed in the cannabis "beat," we exchanged stories of our bouts with mental health issues as if we were talking about the weather. After that initial coffee date when we both actively and unabashedly engaged in what many might consider oversharing, we became not only colleagues at the *Georgia Straight* but also fast friends (who probably annoyed the hell out of our colleagues). We have a lot in common: a passion for writing, an affinity for cannabis, a serious obsession with tattoos, and a feeling that talking about our mental health battles might make them easier for us, and others, to overcome.

"I've been dealing with anxiety and depression from a really young age," Courtenay tells me one afternoon after we sneak away from our cubicles to a more private place to talk. Childhood trauma forced her to grow up a lot more quickly than her peers, she says, exposing her to high levels of stress early in life.

"But when I was twenty-one, I had an abortion—and that was kind of the emotional earthquake that unearthed a lot of mental health issues." Combined with the struggles of living in an unfamiliar city where she had few friends and was in a relationship that seemed to be hanging by a thread, the abortion sent her into a deep depression while kicking her ongoing battle with anxiety into high gear and eventually leading to what psychologists refer to as a dysregulated nervous system.

"It means I can't really pull myself back from extremes," she says.

For Courtenay, these extremes can involve feelings of intense angst that can bring about panic and anxiety attacks, as well as feelings of withdrawal and social anxiety when she's around people. At the height of her struggle, panic attacks occurred often and her feeling of loneliness was all-consuming.

One day, friends began discussing the nuances of medical marijuana at a barbecue, and she listened carefully as one chimed in to say it helped relieve his anxiety. He explained the differences between strains, detailing the characteristics of THC and CBD, and breaking down the science of the endo-cannabinoid system. This helped her get used to the idea of using cannabis before diving right in, and soon enough, any hesitation she had melted away. She began exploring cannabis not as a solution to her anxiety, but as a tool to help her overcome it. Combined with things like conventional therapy, alternative coping mechanisms, and lots and lots of self-love, it has helped keep Courtenay anxiety-attack-free for months on end. With the help of a friend, she conducted her own experiments until, through trial and error, she found the right strains for her anxiety.

"I learned quickly that there are some strains that work better than others," she says, noting that some strains with a higher THC content tended to increase her anxiety, while those that are closer to a one-to-one ratio of THC and CBD were more beneficial.

"The other thing that cannabis does for me is it interrupts the negative thought patterns that occur with anxiety," she says. "Anyone who's suffered with this knows that it tries to pull you back in, and you can try to pull yourself out—but cannabis really helps to bring that relief."

Think of it as a way to gain a bird's-eye view or a refreshed perspective on the issues at hand, she suggests. "It adds a level of rationality that you don't really have when you're having an anxiety attack."

Perpetually Stressed: A Modern Phenomenon?

THESE DAYS, IT'S easy to attribute our pent-up feelings of stress and anxiety to long days at the office, nagging issues in our personal relation-ships, or financial burdens like car repairs or credit card bills. We often look at stress in a negative light: I might blame my anxiety for my inability to function at work, or my stress for my difficulty in settling into peaceful meditation. But when mod-ern humans evolved 200,000 years ago, stress served an entirely different purpose.

While we might foolishly proclaim that hunting for a meal in a grocery store can be stressful, the earth's first humans faced a much more justified sense of stress from competing with other humans and predators for food—not to mention the very real danger of being hunted themselves. Although the causes behind stress and anxiety felt by modern humans and our ancient counterparts are vastly different, the brain's response is identical.

In the 1920s, medical researcher Hans Selye adopted the word "stress" to describe a physical or psychological strain on the human body. He was the first to argue that stress can have an impact on one's health. His model explains that the body responds to stress in three stages: (1) alarm, (2) resistance, and (3) exhaustion. Stage one occurs when the body encounters a threat, or stressor, and reacts with a fight-or-flight response. The sympathetic nervous system is activated when the brain, particularly the amygdala, senses stress and sends a signal to the hypothalamus, which then signals the pituitary and adrenal glands to secrete hormones like adrenaline and cortisol. If the secretion of these hormones doesn't induce homeostasis, it will move to the next stage. During stage two, resistance, the body attempts to return to normal levels of physiological function while cortisol and adrenalin continue to circulate. As this is happening, the parasympathetic nervous system is also trying to return the body to stasis, or a state of balance. This stage is often referred to as chronic stress: cortisol levels remain high, but the body is still able to cope. The final stage of Selye's model, exhaustion, occurs when a stressor exceeds the body's capacity for stress, eventually exhausting its physical resources and rendering the person affected susceptible to disease, and even death.

Anxiety, though closely related, isn't the same thing as stress. While stress is the body's response to an existing stressor and can result in myriad feelings like anger, sadness, or worry, anxiety occurs in the absence of a stressor and is associated primarily with fear and apprehension.

Sometimes it's easy to identify the causes of anxiety; other times, it comes flying out of left field. Though most people experience anxiety in waves, being in a state of perpetual anxiety is like leaving your fight-or-flight response switched on indefinitely. If not addressed, that prolonged effect can contribute to the development of anxiety disorders that can make carrying on with normal life seem next to impossible. Generalized anxiety disorder, panic disorder, social anxiety disorder, obsessive-compulsive disorder, PTSD, and specific phobias all fit under the anxiety umbrella.

However you define them, stress and anxiety are a significant, and growing, problem. The Anxiety and Depression Association of America (ADAA) reports that 18 percent of the population suffers from anxiety disorders,[1] while the American Psychological Association (APA) says nearly a quarter of Americans experience extreme stress on a regular basis.[2]

Historical Use of Cannabis for Anxiety

WHILE THE PHENOMENON of feeling perpetually stressed out by non-life-threatening factors might be a relatively new one, the use of cannabis as a remedy for stress and anxiety could be described as ancient.

In *Marijuana Medicine: A World Tour of the Healing and Visionary Powers of Cannabis*, ethno-pharmacological researcher Christian Rätsch writes that cannabis was used as early as 3000 BCE for this very purpose. It was even referred to in Sumerian texts as "the plant for forgetting worries." Granted, cannabis was consumed in some very different ways then than it is now, but the reasons for using it remain the same.

Today, I might use cannabis to relieve stress and anxiety by enjoying a few puffs from a vaporizer or taking a bath with a THC-infused bath bomb, but in ancient India, a popular way to combat stress involved using a preparation called *bhang*, a paste made from cannabis buds and leaves that was then mixed with milk, ghee, and spices to create a drink. It was often used to facilitate meditation and transcendence. In the sacred Hindu scripture *Atharva Veda* (1400 BCE), cannabis is described as being one of five plants that provide "freedom from distress." *Bhang* is still used today, and is such an integral part of Hindu practices that it was excluded from the government's *Narcotic Drugs and Psychotropic Substances Act* of 1985.

It wasn't until 1843 that cannabis was introduced to Western medicine. William O'Shaughnessy was working in Calcutta when he first witnessed cannabis medicine in action. He soon found himself embracing the plant, using it as a treatment for a number of conditions and consulting with contemporary Indian scholars on the best preparation methods. Eventually O'Shaughnessy discovered that cannabis tinctures were an effective treatment for cholera, and that idea caught the attention of desperate clinicians in Europe and North America who had been unable to find a cure for the fatal disease.

That in turn sparked the interest of even more doctors and scientists, and over the next twenty years, researchers in the Western world published more than a hundred articles about cannabis and its therapeutic values. In 1851, the *U.S. Pharmacopeia* first listed *extractum cannabis*, or cannabis extract, as a recognized medicine. It was included in every subsequent edition until 1942, after the *Marihuana Tax Act* of 1937 made cannabis federally illegal. Similarly, the *Dispensatory of the United States of America*, a guidebook of sorts that listed botanical drugs and their various uses, made claims that cannabis could "compose nervous disquietude," and specifically recommended its use for a host of mental health-related conditions including hysteria, depression, and even insanity.

How Cannabis Can Help

RESEARCHERS TODAY ARE working to piece together how cannabis works in the body to alleviate anxiety. The resulting studies to date have demonstrated that cannabis and its most commonly investigated compounds, the cannabinoids THC and CBD, can modulate anxiety on a dose-dependent basis. But in order to understand how these cannabinoids function relative to the body's stress response, we must first understand the systems that exist regardless of cannabis use or presence.

The endocannabinoid system, or ECS, is a major regulatory system that exists in every mammal. It initiates both psychological and physiological changes as our bodies adapt to new environments or circumstances—think of stress as just another circumstance that our bodies are constantly trying to adapt to. Stress and anxiety will activate a healthy ECS so that it produces endocannabinoids—that is, the cannabinoids in our bodies—as needed. These endocannabinoids then activate the endocannabinoid receptors found throughout our bodies to facilitate the necessary response. In 2012, a team of German researchers completed a study, published in the *Journal of Psychopharmacology*, that showed that endocannabinoid signaling may ensure an appropriate reaction to stressful events, and referred to the ECS as "a regulatory buffer system for emotional response."[3]

A common metaphor often used by scientists compares the ECS to a system of locks and keys: once the key (cannabinoid) is fitted into its corresponding lock (cannabinoid receptor), a chemical message is unlocked and triggers a change in the body that helps us adapt to stress. If we look at this in terms of Selye's stress model, the ECS is very much at play during the resistance stage, when the body is trying to adapt to a persistent source of stress.

Even before researchers were able to illustrate the relationship between anxiety and the ECS, they were well aware that stress and anxiety were among the most common reasons cannabis users gave for consuming the plant. A Canadian study that examined the use of cannabis for therapeutic purposes among a group of 628 people found that 79 percent of respondents used cannabis to relieve their anxiety.[4] A review article in 2017 corroborated that claim with eight cross-sectional studies that came to the same conclusion: relief of anxiety is a primary reason for cannabis use.[5]

Now that we know how the body produces its own cannabinoids to combat stress, it's easier to grasp the way cannabis-derived cannabinoids work in our bodies. Of course, you might be wondering why cannabis is even necessary if our bodies already make their own cannabinoids. Because endocannabinoids are produced on demand and not stored, they can run out if the body is put under so much stress that it exhausts its capacity to create more. When this happens, the ECS becomes unbalanced. (A more detailed explanation of endo-cannabinoids and their receptors can be found in Appendix 1.)

An unbalanced ECS can cause problems, especially when it comes to mental health. In 2014, researchers at Vanderbilt University were able to confirm that when people suffered chronic stress or severe emotional trauma, they were at risk of a reduction in their endocannabinoid production,[6] which subsequently increased their chances of experiencing anxiety. This is where the cannabinoids from cannabis can come in handy. The same study found that when users who were deficient in endocannabinoids consumed cannabis, their anxiety was reduced. You see, THC and CBD act in a similar fashion to the body's endocannabinoids, meaning they can unlock or fit into cannabinoid receptors in the same way. At a neurochemical level, consuming cannabinoids like THC and CBD can help to regulate the body's ECS by working to restore balance. As we mentioned earlier, though, the dosage level plays a large part: too much cannabis, it turns out, disrupts the ECS and can *increase* anxiety.

Finding the line between increasing and decreasing one's anxiety with cannabis has a lot to do with the characteristics of the plant's dominant compounds. We know from the previous chapter that THC is the cannabinoid responsible for the euphoria, or high, that comes with consuming cannabis, and for many first-time users, this feeling isn't always pleasant—in fact, some blame it for making them feel *more* anxious. CBD, however, doesn't cause euphoria. This fact alone has some convinced that CBD might be more effective than THC at treating anxiety.

Cannabis has been shown, over and over in laboratory settings, to be good at regulating anxiety. A 2010 review of the therapeutic use of cannabinoids looked at almost one hundred animal and human studies to determine the potential of the ECS to help treat psychiatric conditions. Scientists wrote that, due to its lack of intoxicating or cognitive effects and its relative safety, "CBD is possibly the cannabinoid more likely to have initial findings translated into clinical practice."[7] The same study also suggested that while THC has been shown to have sedative and sleep-promoting properties, it would be worthwhile to conduct a "careful exploration of the beneficial effects of the association of THC and CBD." Overall, the review found the ECS to be "a promising target for novel therapeutic interventions" in psychiatric conditions, including anxiety.

When we consider the individual qualities of each cannabinoid, another factor that can affect the potency of a compound is its interaction with another compound. Scientists have known since 1974 that CBD can interfere with the desired (and sometimes not-so-desired) effects of THC,[8] and they confirmed in a 1982 study that a dose of CBD could effectively combat side effects of anxiety caused by consuming a dose of THC.[9] (This is why a budtender might advise someone who is feeling unwell after consuming THC to consume a product high in CBD.)

While the 2010 study mentioned earlier suggested that CBD might make a better starting point for patients suffering from anxiety, more recent studies of the literature on the ECS and anxiety take a broader approach, including studies specific to PTSD. The biggest differentiation between individuals with anxiety disorders and individuals with PTSD is that individuals with PTSD form what scientists call a "fear memory," or fear conditioning, after a traumatic event. This can cause flashbacks, aggression, depression, increased heart rate, muscle tension, and insomnia, among other things. PTSD also involves a failure of the normal fear extinction process, meaning that certain reminders, or "triggers," of a traumatic experience can cause conditioned fear responses long after the experience has ended.

Animal studies have shown that enhanced endocannabinoid signaling has an effect on fear memory, with doses of both THC and CBD showing an ability to impair it. One human study found that administering a low dose of THC to healthy subjects helped to modulate the circuits in the brain involved in fear extinction. It notes that the body's endocannabinoid system could very well serve as a "promising target" for PTSD intervention.[10]

Another study that examined the effects of THC on the brain found that THC enhanced functional connectivity between various regions of the amygdala and prefrontal cortex,[11] suggesting that, in the context of a threat, THC can modulate reactivity, potentially reducing our threat perception or enhancing our socio-emotional regulation. Simply put, THC could help us react more appropriately when we're faced with something frightening.

Using Cannabis to Treat Stress and Anxiety

EVIDENCE HAS SHOWN that the difference between reducing one's anxiety with cannabis and accidently increasing it lies in the dose. (Enter a dispensary and you'll hear this saying at least once: "Start low and go slow.") In a 2017 study of the neuropsychiatric effects of cannabis, the researchers write that the high that comes with consuming cannabis "can be achieved with doses of THC as low as 2.5 milligrams in an herbal cigarette and includes a feeling of intoxication, with decreased anxiety, alertness, depression and tension and increased sociability."[12] Another study, looking only at CBD, found that doses between 300 and 600 milligrams reduced anxiety induced in a lab setting, but didn't seem to affect baseline anxiety levels. However, those doses did reduce baseline anxiety in patients with seasonal affective disorder. This study's authors wrote that preclinical evidence "conclusively demonstrates CBD's efficacy in reducing anxiety behaviors relevant to multiple disorders," including the anxiety disorders listed earlier in this chapter.[13]

Now consider that despite these and other studies that note the body's positive response to cannabis in times of stress and anxiety, physicians in many U.S. states aren't permitted to recommend cannabis as a treatment for anxiety disorders. Most states provide physicians with a list of conditions and symptoms that are deemed eligible for treatment with cannabis. The physical health conditions and symptoms tend to be limited to chronic pain, wasting syndrome, nausea, and seizures; the mental health conditions tend to include only PTSD. Only a few states allow doctors to suggest cannabis for other persistent medical conditions.

Dr. Jeremy Spiegel is a physician at Casco Bay Medical in Massachusetts, where he is allowed to exercise his judgment when treating patients whose conditions aren't included in the state's list. He says 25 to 30 percent of his patients use medical cannabis to treat mental health conditions and mood disorders that are often closely related to stress and anxiety. But even when patients have access to the state system and are using cannabis with his approval, Spiegel says, administering cannabis as a treatment for stress- and anxiety-related conditions comes with a unique set of challenges.

Cannabis has more than two hundred active compounds, many of which have yet to be studied, making it unlike any single-molecule medication one might take to treat a given condition, as most drugs contain just one compound. Spiegel says the difference between using cannabis and using a prescription drug can be compared to the difference between eating whole foods and "eating out of a can."

Consider Marinol, a synthetic version of THC that was first approved by the FDA in 1985 and is often administered to patients suffering from side effects associated with chemotherapy, like nausea. Spiegel says that while it might seem logical to draw the conclusion that synthetic THC works in the same way that cannabis-derived THC does, it simply isn't true. When cannabis-derived THC enters the body, it works in conjunction with other cannabinoids and terpenes, some of which can also have anxiety-reducing effects. (The entourage effect mentioned earlier.) Terpenes are powerful organic compounds that exist in a variety of plants and are responsible for giving them their unique aromas. It's currently thought that there are over one hundred in cannabis, including notably stress-relieving terpenes like linalool (which smells like lavender), myrcene (found in mango), and limonene (which has an aroma profile similar to citrus's). While Spiegel recognizes the clinical importance of studying each individual compound, he says that administering them individually will never produce the same results as consuming the plant in its whole form. This makes cannabis treatment exciting, but also more difficult to control.

Spiegel refrains from making any recommendations about which strains or cannabinoid ratios to use for stress and anxiety, but he does tell patients to keep an open mind when they're visiting their local dispensary, where budtenders help patients identify which products might work best. He says patients who don't want to get high often ask about CBD products, but he reminds them that while CBD does offer benefits on its own, a patient who uses it exclusively can build up a tolerance to the compound that will require them to eventually increase their dose. Patients may find that if they are using a medicine containing a single compound, they build up a tolerance more quickly. (This can get expensive, as products made exclusively with CBD tend to be more costly.) When that occurs, he'll recommend that patients introduce THC in the form of a balanced tincture, capsule, or strain to offset the body's tolerance to CBD.

Depending on where you live, accessing cannabis to treat mild to moderate stress and anxiety might be as simple as popping into a dispensary, but choosing the right product might be more challenging. The differences between varieties of cannabis and each person's ECS mean that there is no such thing as a one-size-fits-all solution. A budtender might suggest that a person dealing with high stress and anxiety lean toward a sedating strain like Death Bubba or Granddaddy Purple, which are both THC-dominant strains known to relax the mind while creating a peaceful body high. Of course, the patient might prefer a strain like Cannatonic, which is a CBD-dominant strain with a small amount of THC that is often recommended for anxiety. (Based on what we know about THC's ability to increase anxiety in high doses, this might be a safe place to start.)

Inhalation is recommended if you're looking for a quick onset of relief from stress. If smoking isn't something you're interested in taking up, vaporizing might be for you. (Vaporizers also make for a more discreet solution to a midday bout with anxiety than a big, smelly joint.) Other options like tinctures and edibles provide a different set of benefits because their effects tend to last much longer. Tinctures and oils are available in specific ratios of THC to CBD, like 1:1, 1:2, or 1:4, and some manufacturers have created products for different times of day. For example, a daytime tincture or oil might be made with more CBD than THC so that users don't experience the high associated with THC during the day, while an evening tincture might be formulated with higher levels of THC. Other options include capsules, which are made from liquid cannabis extractions and don't feel much different than taking conventional medication. Whatever your preference, most cannabis experts agree that whole-plant medicine, rather than products made with isolated compounds, will always offer users a more flexible treatment experience, no matter the ailment.

3
...

BOOSTING MOOD AND CREATIVITY

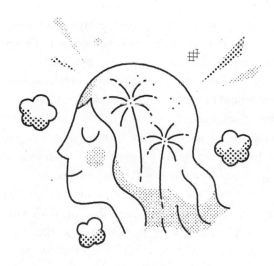

Case Study: Jon Bent

FROM AN OUTSIDER'S perspective, one might conclude that Jon Bent's role as a grower of medical cannabis doesn't require a whole lot of creativity. But according to the twenty-year veteran cultivator, that would be incorrect. For Bent, a creative mind who spent much of his youth drawing and reading comic books, not only does cannabis deserve credit for helping him gain a stronger ability to focus, it's also given him a more positive outlook on life.

By phone from Winnipeg, Bent tells me that for most of his life he's been dealing with what he describes as "excess mental energy" that leads to jumbled thoughts, a lack of motivation, and a floating anxiety that is often hard to ignore. At age seventeen, he began experiencing thoughts he describes as "counterproductive and unimportant," and that left him lacking confidence in his creative ability and struggling to focus on certain tasks. But when he began using cannabis, he experienced a return to baseline that allowed him to think more clearly.

"I've used the analogy before to describe it as almost like a melting pot on the stove, with a whole bunch of fragmented thoughts and nothing really binding or forming production," he tells me. "But when I use cannabis, my thoughts bind together, I'm confident and productive, and good thoughts come out of all that mumbo-jumbo excess."

For the last several years, cannabis has been Bent's go-to solution. Before that, as a young adult while working the night shift at a local bus depot, Bent's racing mind kept him from sleeping, adding insomnia to his mental frustration. His doctor advised he try an antidepressant—Zoloft—to help regulate his mood and untamed thoughts.

"It was a very heavy SSRI at the time, but I tried it for a bit, and I remember thinking, 'Wow, this is like MDMA,'" he recalls. Feeling both overpowered and numbed by the drug, he realized that Zoloft alone wouldn't address his problem. "It's like when an athlete gets a shot of cortisone," he says. "It never really gets to the root of the pain. You might feel good, and for a bit, you might even feel on top of the world, but when it wears off, you haven't dealt with the problem."

As you'll learn later in this chapter, mood and creativity are closely linked. While Bent admits he's not doing the creative things he was doing as a teen, smoking cannabis allows him to have a better handle on his tasks as a grower and breeder of cannabis plants—a job he says allows for *some* creativity—while also lifting his spirits. He recalls his first venture into entrepreneurship: opening the first of what would eventually be three hydroponics stores was a big undertaking from the self-proclaimed "small farm guy," and he says he often experienced negative thoughts brought on by the stress of running a small business. Using cannabis to overcome that stress has served him well, and over the years, he's made many friends who share his appreciation for the way cannabis can tame the mind.

"I know quite a few people that are entrepreneurial and really passionate, always on the go, and they all seem to agree that cannabis really helps channel all that energy into a good thing, and feelings that are positive."

Mood, Creativity, and Where They Intersect

NO ONE'S IMMUNE to foul moods. Maybe you failed an exam, or perhaps it was something less serious, like spilling your coffee or getting stuck in traffic. Whatever the case, moods caused by everyday triggers can be nasty, and they often derail our plans for an otherwise productive day. Thankfully, humans have developed coping skills to prevent us from getting stuck in a funk that might otherwise lead to a bad week, or even a bad month. However, while we all experience a bad mood every now and then, if we find ourselves feeling down in the dumps for extended periods of time we might run the risk of being in the throes of something far more serious than a mood swing.

A bad mood might leave you feeling depressed for a day or two, but a mood disorder could leave you feeling depressed for months, even years. Recent statistics have shown the number of people falling victim to mood disorders is growing: in Canada, the prevalence of mood disorders rose from 7.9 percent in 2015 to 8.4 percent in 2016.[1] In the United States, mood disorders are slightly more common, with 9.5 percent of the population affected.[2]

People experiencing mood disorders might lose interest in their daily activities, avoid social situations, lose their appetite, experience low energy levels, and have difficulty falling or staying asleep. They might also experience episodes of severe depression or mania, as well as erratic moods that leave them feeling like a million bucks at one moment and completely worthless the next.

Beyond just affecting our perception of things or our productivity, a particular mood can also affect our creativity. This can be critical for people working in fields like writing, design, or music. But before we can understand where mood and creativity intersect, let's break down the origins of creative thought, and how psychologists separate it from other ways of thinking.

While studying intelligence in the 1950s, psychologist Joy Paul Guilford first coined the terms *divergent thinking* and *convergent thinking* to describe the two distinct thought processes that humans use to problem-solve. Say you're asked to calculate the tip on a bill at lunch. If you were to calculate the tax manually, you'd use what Guilford referred to as convergent thinking. This refers to a systematic, logical thought process that results in a single solution. Creativity isn't relevant to convergent thinking—you don't need creativity to answer questions like "What's the capital of Japan?" or "What's the speed limit here?" Divergent thinking, on the other hand, is considered more spontaneous and free-flowing. It's the kind of thinking we do when we're presented with an abstract problem that could have more than one solution, like what we want to wear, or how we could prepare a certain food item.

Decades of research have shown that mood can have a direct effect on creativity. Though the relationship is complex, significant data shows a correlation: multiple studies indicate that a positive mood can enhance creativity. One such study published in 2008 showed that creativity was enhanced by "positive mood states that are activating," like happiness. (If happiness is activating, a deactivating mood state might be feeling relaxed.) While a negative mood resulting in feelings of sadness didn't seem to affect creativity at all, negative moods that resulted in activating feelings like fear or anxiety resulted in lower creativity.[3] The artists who are reading—not just the painters, but the writers, producers, surgeons, and all the other modern-day problem solvers—will know all too well how mood affects their ability to produce quality work from one day to the next. Understanding the correlation between mood and creativity helps us make sense of how cannabis can come into play in both areas.

Historical Use of Cannabis for Mood and Creativity

WHILE IT'S NOT uncommon to hear of cannabis being used in a therapeutic sense to help stomp out a bad mood or to promote creative thought, early historical evidence of cannabis being used for these purposes is a little less plentiful than it is for cannabis being used as a pain reliever or sleep aid.

The earliest record of cannabis use in a medicinal context dates back to 2737 BCE, when Emperor Shen Nung of China lauded cannabis

and its derivatives for their ability to treat everything from gout to rheumatism and constipation to
"absent-mindedness." It's likely that the emperor,
the Father of Chinese Medicine who is credited with
the discovery of plant medicines such as cannabis,
ephedra, and ginseng, felt the elevating effects
of cannabis on his mood: one excerpt from the
Shennong Ben Cao Jing, the world's oldest pharmacopeia based on spoken traditions passed down
from the emperor, describes cannabis as something
that "lightens one's body." We learned in Chapter
2 that the ancient Hindu scripture *Atharva Veda*
refers to cannabis as a plant that provides "freedom
from distress," and while this certainly implies that
cannabis is an effective anxiolytic, "distress" also
refers to sorrow and sadness, so it's not a stretch to
assume that its properties as a mood enhancer were
also popular in India.

In *The Encyclopedia of Psychoactive Plants:
Ethnopharmacology and Its Applications*, author
Christian Rätsch quotes a leader of the Rastafari in
Jamaica. There, cannabis is used as religious sacra-
ment, but also to "overcome illness, suffering and
death."[4] In a more general sense, he says it's also
used as a therapeutic way to promote "comfort"—a
word that invokes the idea of overcoming a state
of unease, pain, or grief. A much earlier report of
cannabis being used as an antidepressant comes
from Dr. Jacques-Joseph Moreau's 1845 publication,

Hashish and Mental Illness. Hashish was the drug of choice among France's intellectual elite in the nineteenth century, and Moreau was a dedicated member of Paris's Club des Hashischins, where men like Victor Hugo and Alexandre Dumas would smoke hashish, a form of cannabis resin, with the intention of discovering the benefits of drug intoxication. In his book, Moreau wrote that using hashish created "a feeling of gaiety and joy inconceivable to those who have never experienced it."[5]

Early historical evidence of cannabis being used for reasons of creativity is even more difficult to nail down, but if we consider the way Shen Nung used it to "communicate with spirits," or the way Parisian intellectuals flocked to the Club des Hashischins to engage with art and each other under the influence of Egyptian hashish, I think it's fair to say that the human race has always been curious about the herb's ability to open the mind and spur imagination. We see further evidence of this from the Assyrians of ancient Mesopotamia, who thought using cannabis as incense could promote inspiration and spiritual visions.[6] Even William Shakespeare, one of the world's greatest dramatists, is thought to have used cannabis. This is the conclusion South African scientists came to in 2001 when they discovered traces of cannabis in clay tobacco pipes at Shakespeare's residence in Stratford-upon-Avon. While it's certainly a controversial point that most academics will contend with, not least because of Shakespeare's love of word play, the Bard does mention "a noted weed" in Sonnet 76. Some believe he is referring to cannabis.

In more recent years, many creatives have come out of the "weedwork," so to speak, crediting cannabis for its ability to spur their creativity in even the darkest of times. From Louis Armstrong, Chuck Berry, Jerry Garcia, and Willie Nelson to more modern artists like Alanis Morissette, Lady Gaga, Miley Cyrus, and Jay-Z—who famously proclaimed about one of his most popular songs, "I smoked some weed, and that's how I finished 'Izzo'"—many musicians are huge proponents of cannabis use for the purpose of generating new music. The same goes for writers like Hunter S. Thompson, Maya Angelou, and Stephen King. Comedians, actors, chefs, and other professionals in the public eye who rely on their creative impetus to bring home the bacon have come forward to say that cannabis has a distinct influence on how they operate—for the better.

How Cannabis Can Help

WHEN CONSIDERING THE historical and present-day use of cannabis to both regulate moods and spur creativity, it's safe to say that there is plenty of anecdotal evidence to support the idea that cannabis can be useful for some people. But what about scientific evidence? Dr. Zach Walsh is a registered clinical psychologist, researcher, and instructor at the University of British Columbia (UBC) in Kelowna, B.C., where he has studied the effects of cannabis on the human psyche for nearly a decade. Walsh says he has no doubt that cannabis has the potential to alter one's mood and improve the symptoms of an ongoing mood disorder.

"If we look across the board at studies of cannabis users, one of the prime motives for use is that it does impact mood," Walsh says. And while he says the exact nature of these effects is debatable, the effects of cannabis are not. For Walsh, to describe the effects of cannabis without mentioning mood would be to miss a critical piece of what cannabis does to a person.

In a 2017 systematic review of medical cannabis and mental health, Walsh and a team of researchers looked at sixty articles published between 1977 and 2015. Key relevant findings from his study show a common theme: in one cross-sectional study, 69 percent of medical cannabis users said that mood was a prominent reason for their use. Another showed that patients who used cannabis said they felt relief from feelings of anxiety, depression, anger, and panic. Several cross-sectional surveys showed that cannabis use for therapeutic purposes can improve mood and well-being among individuals with medical conditions.[7] That is to say, while cannabis may be used with the intention of treating a specific condition like chronic pain or in conjunction with other treatments for cancer, patients also find it useful for lifting their spirits.

"One of the things that's so fascinating to me about cannabis is that it is so hard to actually describe what cannabis does," Walsh says. "What does it feel like?" Because substances like alcohol or antidepressants have a more direct effect on a specific neurotransmitter system in the brain, he says, it's easier to describe their effects: "Alcohol makes you feel sort of loose, antidepressants make you feel tired, but cannabis? It's definitely a lot harder to nail down."

Another area of Walsh's expertise is PTSD. While it's considered by some mental health specialists to be an anxiety disorder, many symptoms of PTSD are closely related to mood—for instance, it causes patients to develop what Walsh calls "a hair trigger," which can lead to irritability and aggression. "One thing that you'll hear patients with PTSD say is that cannabis makes them more tolerable, more tolerant, and generally easier to be around," he says.

That notion is reflected in several studies that are included in Walsh's review, including a cross-sectional study out of New Mexico, where patients who used cannabis therapeutically reported reductions of 75 percent in symptoms of avoidance, hyperarousal, and re-experiencing. But with research on PTSD and other disorders linked to mood still in its infancy, the question remains: What is it about cannabis that means it can have a positive effect on mood?

The answer may lie in the body's endo-cannabinoid system. In a placebo-controlled, cross-sectional study published in 2013, researchers administered THC to fourteen healthy people. By using functional magnetic resonance imaging (fMRI) to measure subjects' brain activity while showing them images of fearful faces, happy faces, and a control image, they found that THC interacted with the brain's emotional content by reducing the brain's negative bias.[8]

"These results suggest that administration of THC shifts the brain's bias for stimuli that have a negative impact toward a bias for stimuli that have a positive impact. Our findings support the hypothesis of involvement of the ECB [endocannabinoid] system in modulation of emotional processing," the study reads. Essentially, subjects who were given THC had lower brain activity when they saw the negative images than subjects who were given a placebo and then shown the same images. That may not sound that impressive, but negativity bias—the phenomenon by which the brain is more sensitive to bad news, events, or feelings—has been linked to mental illnesses including depression and anxiety.

So if THC has the ability to make us less suscep-tible to negativity, why aren't more people using it? This is probably something experienced cannabis users have asked themselves thousands of times, but according to Walsh, there could be downsides to using cannabis for mood regulation too often. "If you're relying on cannabis and you're using it to regulate your mood, you might be impairing yourself in other ways that could detract from your quality of life," he says. "The same things that can help with your mood might adversely affect your cognitive function, and depending on the context, there could be some problems."

Walsh says that people who become depen-dent on cannabis might become irritable when they withdraw from it, but he says it's important to remember that other, more accepted substances—like caffeine—can have the same effect. "In that way, it's really no different from coffee. If someone's reli-ant on caffeine and they don't have their morning coffee, they're irritable! ... [Cannabis] is like cof-fee, in the sense that people can be addicted to it, if we want to use that term, or have a dependence on it, and that doesn't necessarily interfere with their functioning." Context, Walsh says, is every-thing. "People say, 'cannabis can be addictive,' and the question is, in what context? Saying something is addictive without talking about the consequences of that addiction can be misleading, because we have all these associations with the term 'addiction,' without really thinking of the many things that we're addicted to."

If you thought the scientific data backing up the link between cannabis use and mood was slim, know that the research linking cannabis use with creativity is even slimmer. A study conducted in 2014 by a group of Dutch scientists tried to determine whether cannabis had an effect on creativity by administering different doses of vaporized cannabis to three groups. One group received a low dose of THC—5.5 milligrams—a second received a high dose—22 milligrams—and a third group received a placebo. They found that, while "cannabis users often claim that cannabis has the potential to enhance their creativity," those who were subjected to the higher dose of THC performed poorly when asked to perform tasks requiring divergent thinking. The less potent cannabis did not seem to enhance or hinder the divergent thought processes of those who received it. "The frequently reported feeling of heightened creativity could be an illusion," conclude the scientists, suggesting that smoking a joint might not be the best way to overcome writer's block, and that smoking several "might actually be counter-productive."[9]

As someone who used cannabis to overcome writer's block at many different points as I wrote this book, I respectfully disagree—and I'm sure many readers will too. What if the people in the above sample weren't creative people? It's a question I asked myself before I spoke with Dr. Carrie Cuttler, a psychology professor from Washington State University, who has been studying cannabis use and the psyche for many years. When I bring up the subject of creativity, she says it's a topic not often discussed in the context of cannabis. At the time of our discussion, she was reviewing a paper by one of her graduate students, Emily LaFrance, who was asking a question that had less to do with the acute effects of cannabis on creativity and more to do with the personality traits of cannabis users.

In conducting research ahead of their study, "Inspired by Mary Jane? Mechanisms Underlying Enhanced Creativity in Cannabis Users," Cuttler tells me that the previous literature on the effects of cannabis on creativity comes to different conclusions than the study that deemed heightened creativity by cannabis use "an illusion": "It suggested to us that low doses of THC seem to enhance divergent thinking, relative to a placebo," she says, noting that findings are often inconsistent. "There are also several studies that show absolutely no effects of THC on divergent thinking, while others still say THC actually perturbs divergent thinking."

Because Cuttler and LaFrance were not allowed to give people cannabis in the college laboratory, they had to frame their question in a different way, instead asking, "Are cannabis users as people more creative?" Taking two groups (one of nonusers and one of cannabis users, but both sober) and administering a self-report and a series of psychological tests, they found that not only did cannabis users report having higher levels of creativity, they actually performed better than nonusers on tests of convergent thinking, something that came as a surprise to Cuttler. "We didn't find anything significant on divergent thinking, but what is really interesting is what we found when we looked at personality difference within cannabis users and nonusers," she says. "One of the differences was that cannabis users are more open to experience, and openness to experience is moderately related to creativity." She says when the variable for openness to experience was removed, all of the differences between cannabis users and nonusers relating to creativity—both self-reported and objective—disappeared.[10] "What this suggests is that yes, cannabis users are more creative than nonusers, but it's because they are more open to experience."

Using Cannabis for Mood and Creativity

WHILE THE USE of cannabis for mood-related reasons is common, it's also highly subjective and deeply personal: A cannabis product that might make me feel like I'm on top of the world could induce panic in another. Similarly, something that might make me feel like a creative genius could make someone else feel like they're overdue for a long nap. It's why almost every expert I spoke with on this subject was hesitant about recommending a specific compound, strain, or method of ingestion: the compounds in cannabis affect everyone differently, because our endocannabinoid systems are all different. We already know that there is certainly no one-size-fits-all solution for mood disorders or overcoming interruptions to our creative process, and that is especially true when it comes to cannabis.

Before picking out which compound ratio or terpene profile might serve you best in the midst of a mood swing or a creative block, it's important to consider both your current state and what effect you're looking for. Are you feeling sad, angry, or low? Do your mood swings bring up unnecessary bouts of anxiety? What if you want to feel better, but you don't want to get high? Considering what we know about the therapeutic compounds THC, which can help alter our negative bias toward a situation, and CBD, which has been shown to have anxiolytic, or calming, properties and doesn't come with the intoxicating effects of THC, narrowing down choices becomes a little easier.

Another question worth asking yourself is whether the relief you're looking for needs to be immediate and short-term or long-lasting. Do you want to feel positive throughout the day, or are you trying to overcome temporary feelings of negativity? Answering this question will help you determine which method of consumption will provide the best relief for your situation. Where smoking or vaporizing might take you from negative to positive within a few minutes, consuming a small dose in tincture or capsule form in the morning, afternoon, and evening can promote lasting feelings of positivity.

While Jon Bent, the man featured in the case study at the beginning of this chapter, told me he preferred to smoke strains with a one-to-one ratio of THC to CBD for quick delivery and a balanced return to his baseline mental state, I've spoken with a few artists and designers who prefer to avoid euphoria. They stick with products high in CBD to be at their most "organic," if you will, while creating. A close friend who paints enjoys putting a teaspoon of CBD-infused honey into his tea. Another likes to vaporize a high-CBD strain before sitting down to start her next project. And while some research might suggest that high doses of THC may not benefit the creative process, there are *absolutely* people out there who feed off the "stoned" feeling that comes with the consumption of a high-THC product. I've known dozens of musicians and audiophiles who enjoy hitching a ride on

THC-induced waves of euphoria as they write new songs or sample new beats. If you're feeling conflicted, it's worth mentioning that research in this area, though improving in its quality, is minimal, and often conducted in a way that is biased against cannabis users. But as cannabis use becomes more and more popular—even legal in some parts of the world—these biases are slowly being shed.

4

. . .

METABOLISM,
WEIGHT MANAGEMENT,
AND EXERCISE
RECOVERY

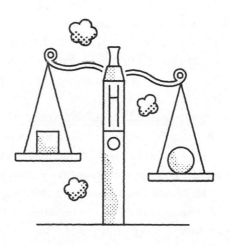

Case Study: Ross Rebagliati
. . . .

IN 1998, I was too young to make sense of why it occurred, but I can vaguely recall the drama in the news when Ross Rebagliati, a Canadian snowboarder from my hometown of Vancouver, B.C., had his Olympic gold medal taken away because he tested positive for THC. (Luckily, the medal was later returned, and eventually the Olympic threshold for THC increased.) It wasn't until I watched Robin Williams's *Live on Broadway* special, in which he joked about the redundancy of testing snowboarders for cannabis, that it all made sense to me. "Marijuana enhances many things, colors, tastes, sensations, but you are certainly not fucking empowered," Williams joked. "The only way it's a performance-enhancing drug is if there's a big fucking Hershey bar at the end of the run."[1] As funny as I still find the joke, it plays into a stereo-type that Rebagliati doesn't necessarily agree with.

These days, he's deeply embedded in Canada's burgeoning cannabis industry and lives with his family in Kelowna, B.C., but in the years leading up to his gold medal win at the 1998 Winter Olympics in Nagano, Japan, he lived in Whistler, B.C., argu-ably one of the world's greatest destinations for winter sports.

"I moved up there from Vancouver in 1990, and that's when I ran into a bunch of backcountry ski-ers and professional mountain bikers at the top of their game—like, the best in the world—all using cannabis, all day long," he tells me by phone. It's hard to stop myself from grinning as he recalls his initial reaction to the idea that professional ath-letes could actually use cannabis to become better at their sport. "I had never thought of it in that way before, because in 1990, there was no Inter-net, and we didn't know anything—except that we liked it."

He describes using cannabis each morning "with coffee and toast" at 5 a.m.—rising well before his friends who had spent the night drinking—and getting up the mountain early for the best runs, taking breaks in between to refuel, drink water, and smoke another joint. "It was then that I realized that it kind of takes your mind off the enormity of the task that you're trying to do and helps you break

THE LITTLE BOOK OF CANNABIS

down the situation, feel the equipment, and be in tune with your environment," he says.

I quip that his dedication to rising at the crack of dawn (in the winter, no less) completely obliterates the idea of the dopey snowboarder who uses cannabis. And with a chuckle and a few "eh's" for emphasis, Rebagliati reiterates that it was those who opted for alcohol the night before that didn't make it up the mountain until 11 a.m. Those who chose cannabis? They slept well, had great runs, and later experienced relief from their aches and pains after a long day on the mountain.

At forty-seven, he says using cannabis for almost thirty years has helped him maintain a healthy lifestyle by encouraging a balanced diet and lots of exercise. Though he might feel a few more aches and pains than he did at twenty-seven, he says cannabis still helps him fight inflammation and discomfort from a previous day's workout, while also helping him sleep through the night and maintain a positive attitude during the day. He says that the benefits of using it have trickled down into every aspect of his life, and he describes his use as "one huge good decision." He says, "I have gravitated toward using cannabis every day, and not consuming as much alcohol because of it, and I think, overall, it leads to a better lifestyle."

When I ask whether or not cannabis use affects his ability to manage his weight, Rebagliati jumps at the question: "Cannabis use has been linked to low BMI," he says, "and as it happens, I'm about 5 foot 10 and 190 pounds. I was at 186 pounds at the Olympics twenty years ago, so I guess you could say I've been pretty constant."

Though he consumes products containing both of cannabis's most common compounds, he says athletes should really consider CBD for its anti-inflammatory and anti-anxiety properties. He confidently predicts that CBD will soon become a daily staple of an athlete's diet.

Three Surprising Areas with Potential

IT'S A CULT rumor that Shaggy, the forgetful and perpetually hungry character in the popular cartoon series *Scooby Doo*, is a cannabis user. And Jughead, of the classic *Archie* comics? About as stereotypical a stoner as it gets. Like Shaggy's penchant for sandwiches, Jughead's obsession with cheeseburgers is a classic symptom of "the munchies": the idea that, post–cannabis consumption, one develops a ravenous appetite for unhealthy food. The archetype of the hungry, skinny hippie is repeated in so many pop culture references that it might be hard to imagine a cannabis user's relationship with food as anything other than unhealthy. Thankfully, the increasingly common use and endorsement of cannabis by athletes, fitness enthusiasts, and health experts is smashing the ill-informed notion that excessive cannabis use leads to unwarranted hunger, sluggishness, and weight gain. But before we can understand what new research says about the relationship between cannabis and your waistline, let's break down three areas that scientists agree have huge potential in the context of therapeutic cannabis use.

Metabolism is essentially the process responsible for converting the nutrients in what we consume into the energy required to carry out bodily functions. When energy isn't required, it's stored in the body for later. A person's metabolic rate depends on a number of factors, including but not limited to muscle mass, height and weight, age, genetics, exercise habits, and diet. Later, we'll learn how cannabis can play a role in regulating metabolic rate.

While metabolism is an ongoing physiological process, *weight management* is about trying to stay within a healthy range, ideally by maintaining a healthy diet and level of physical activity. The notion of frequent encounters with "the munchies" might lead you to believe that cannabis has zero value in the context of weight management, but new research suggests that it might play a role in maintaining a healthy body weight.

If you exercise, you'll know that a workout can lead to sore muscles that leave you feeling less than inspired to get up the next day and repeat the same routine. Professional athletes (or athletic enthusiasts with greater personal will than I) who don't have the option of sleeping through a morning regimen rely on different tricks and techniques to speed up their *athletic recovery*, helping them get back in the game more quickly. Some swear by certain supplements, while others rely on strictly regimented sleep schedules, stretching, and ancillary treatments like massage therapy and acupuncture. Today, it's not uncommon to find pro athletes endorsing cannabis start-up companies on their Instagram pages, or blogging about their success with a certain cannabis-based treatment for an injury.

Historical Use of Cannabis for Metabolism, Weight Management, and Exercise Recovery
....

ADMITTEDLY, THE DESIRE to learn more about the effects of cannabis in the context of maintaining a healthy body weight stems from society's modern-day obsession with appearance—something I think we can be fairly certain early cannabis users didn't concern themselves with. While history's cannabis users may not have known it, they likely experienced the same benefits of cannabis use that scientists are only now beginning to understand.

We know that stress and weight gain have a very close relationship: when you experience increased tension or stress, levels of the hormone cortisol begin to rise, potentially leading to overeating and changes in blood sugar that can leave you craving nutritionally poor foods that are high in sugar and fat. We know Shen Nung and the authors of the *Atharva Veda* experienced the relaxing, sleep-enhancing, and pain-reducing effects of cannabis, so it's highly likely they also felt the regulatory effects of the plant's cannabinoids and terpenes on their metabolism and body weight.

How Cannabis Can Help

AS COUNTERINTUITIVE AS it may seem to some, the latest research on the relationship between cannabis use and metabolism indicates a few things. First, the plant has far greater potential as a supplement for weight regulation than previously thought possible; and second, in the broader sense, whether one is aware of the side effect or not, casual cannabis use over time can lead to a more stable body weight and even a smaller waistline. The research on the relationship between cannabis use and metabolism seems to suggest that, despite cannabis users' possibly consuming more calories than nonusers, it doesn't seem to affect their health in an adverse way.

A study published in 2006 by a team of researchers from the Department of Epidemiology and Biostatistics at the University of California came to some surprising conclusions. The CARDIA Study (Coronary Artery Risk Development in Young Adults), a longitudinal study conducted over 15 years with 3,617 participants, found that cannabis users consumed an average of 600 more calories per day than nonusers.[2] While conventional schools of wisdom might have you believe that prolonged increased caloric consumption should ultimately result in an increased body mass index (BMI), researchers found the opposite: not only was use not associated with increased BMI, it also had no association with higher blood lipids or blood sugar levels (risk factors for heart disease) and it didn't lead to an increased rate of cardiovascular disease.

A more recent study on the topic,[3] published by researchers at the University of Miami, went a step further by examining the potential relationship between cannabis and metabolic syndrome, a group of conditions including high blood pressure, high blood sugar, elevated waist circumference, abnormal cholesterol, and abnormal triglyceride levels. When these conditions occur simultaneously, the risk of cardiovascular disease, stroke, and diabetes increases substantially.

"I started studying cannabis in about 2008," says Dr. Denise Vidot, an assistant professor at the

University of Miami and a co-author of the study. "Back then especially, there was hardly anything published on [the association between cannabis and] physical health." The cross-sectional study she and her team published in 2016 analyzed a group of 8,478 people who had completed a series of national health and nutrition surveys between 2005 and 2010. She admits that the idea of the "munchies" played into her initial hypothesis, telling me she figured that cannabis use would be associated with an increased risk of experiencing the five distinct conditions that can lead to metabolic syndrome.

"I would say there were two major surprises to me, and the first was what we found about waist circumference," she says. Dividing the group first by sex to account for different genetic markers among men and women, and then separating each of those groups into never users, past users, and current users of cannabis, Vidot came to some interesting conclusions about the role cannabis might have played in the size of their waistlines. While women who used cannabis showed a slightly smaller average waist circumference than nonusers, men who were current users had a significantly smaller waist circumference (25.5 percent) than those who had never used cannabis.[4]

"In this research, we also found that the prevalence of abnormal glucose levels was lower among current users, and that to me was also surprising," she says. Both current and past users had significantly lower fasting glucose levels than those who had never touched cannabis. (Low fasting glucose is a good thing, because sustained high glucose levels can lead to adverse effects, including diabetes and an increased risk of cardiovascular disease.)

While the study indicated that cannabis users had a lower prevalence of most of the five conditions that contribute to metabolic syndrome, blood pressure seemed to be the exception. Current cannabis users had higher systolic blood pressure than nonusers, although they didn't have higher diastolic blood pressure. (*Systolic pressure* refers to the amount of pressure that blood exerts on arteries while the heart is contracting; *diastolic pressure* refers to the amount of pressure exerted in between beats, when the heart relaxes. Remember this next time you get your blood pressure checked: the systolic pressure is the top number in a blood pressure reading, and the diastolic is the bottom number.)

In the end, Vidot's team concluded that cannabis users were 54 percent less likely to suffer from metabolic syndrome than those who had never used cannabis. While the findings of other studies on the topic seem to be, for the most part, consistent with Vidot's findings on weight management—though they take a slightly different approach, five of eight studies featured in a literature review documenting the association between cannabis use and change in weight came to similar conclusions[5]—she says that in future studies, she'd like to be able to take into account how users actually consume cannabis (whether it is smoked, vaporized, or ingested), as well as their frequency of use. She'd also consider factors like participants' physical health, diet, and level of fitness, which weren't considered in her initial study but probably influenced the results.

While Vidot's work is helpful in indicating whether or not cannabis use affects certain health factors like waist circumference, glucose levels, and blood pressure, it doesn't tell us which compound (or combination of compounds) in the plant is responsible for what appears to be regulation of the body's metabolism. While scientists have made educated guesses, few have actually studied specific compounds in the context of weight management. But with an increased interest in cannabis's ability to regulate body weight, a team of scientists at Daegu University in Korea decided to do exactly that. Their research, published in the journal *Molecular and Cellular Biochemistry* in 2016, highlighted the potential benefits of one compound in particular—the nonintoxicating cannabinoid CBD—in the treatment and prevention of obesity.

In studying the effects of CBD on immature fat cells called preadipocytes, they found that, by stimulating specific genes and proteins, the cannabinoid enhanced the body's ability to break down fat, while decreasing the production of proteins involved in producing fat cells. CBD also promoted "fat browning," where white-colored fat in the body is converted into a more burnable tissue called brown fat, and increased both the number and activity of mitochondria, the cell components that metabolize fuel for energy, enabling the body to burn calories more efficiently.[6]

While CBD has been getting lots of press in the context of many different health considerations including weight control, a much lesser known compound has garnered some attention for the same reason. Tetrahydrocannabivarin, or THCV, is an analogue of THC thought to be about a quarter as potent as its better-known counterpart.[7] A number of studies have suggested that THCV can lead to weight loss, decreased body fat, and increased energy in mice,[8] and scientists have determined that this has much to do with the way it interacts with the body's endocannabinoid system, or ECS. While THCV affects the same receptors in the brain as THC, it acts much differently: THC acts as an agonist, activating the receptor to stimulate hunger, but THCV acts as an antagonist, blocking the receptor and suppressing appetite, or at least halting the appetite-stimulating effect. While both THC and THCV bring about feelings of euphoria, the heady effects of THCV are said to last about half as long as the effects of THC. And where ingesting large amounts of the former might lead to a snack attack, cannabis strains high in THCV will likely lead to less interest in food.

Scientific data on cannabis use in the context of exercise is less widespread than research on metabolism or weight management, though one oft-cited review of the literature published in 2013 does an excellent job of breaking down the way a number of different substances affect athletic performance. In summarizing the few studies that have considered cannabis in this way, the article's authors write, "the ergogenic effects of marijuana are questionable, as its performance enhancing effect, if any, has yet to be established."[9] Some studies included in this literature review, the earliest of which was conducted in 1975, suggested that using cannabis as a sort of preworkout supplement led to acute effects such as elevated heart rate and blood pressure.[10] While grip strength in subjects didn't change, increased heart rate caused by consumption was associated with reduced capacity for physical activity. Another study suggested that a small dose of THC had no effect on blood pressure, ventilation, or oxygen uptake during exercise.[11] While conclusions of the review were mixed, the authors don't completely discount the possibility that cannabis can have some benefit in the context of athletics: "If there is any positive effect of marijuana, it likely only indirectly improves performance," they write.[12] These indirect benefits could include a reduction in precompetition stress and anxiety, greater relaxation, and improved sleep quality, all of which are noted by Ross Rebagliati at the start of this chapter.

A systematic review examining how common the use of cannabis is among athletes found that it was the second-most commonly used substance after alcohol,[13] but also noted methodological flaws in some of the existing literature, including a lack of longitudinal data and an overreliance on convenience samples.

"Surprisingly, marijuana use, although under-reported, is likely common among athletes," the authors write,[14] noting that athletes who do self-report say they use marijuana to "enhance sport performance." While research works to catch up to the anecdotal evidence from professional athletes, including former NFL player Ricky Williams, UFC fighters Nate and Nick Diaz, and former NBA star Kareem Abdul-Jabbar, a whole range of people from casual exercise enthusiasts to dedicated endurance athletes seems curious about how cannabis could play a role in their athletic performance and recovery.

Using Cannabis for a Healthy Body

WHEN WE LOOK at what the research says about cannabis in the context of metabolism and weight management, it seems reasonable to conclude that the positive effects on these areas are a result of ongoing use—more of a stabilization over time than a quick weight loss remedy. A healthier metabolism and more stable body weight may be a side effect of consistent cannabis use, but don't expect to drop five pounds after smoking your first joint.

When you're using cannabis with the intention of amping up your energy ahead of a workout or easing aches and pains in the hours that follow, how you decide to consume cannabis plays a very important role in how you'll feel. Where some athletes swear by gel capsules or oils before a workout because they prefer not to smoke, others enjoy the quick onset of inhalation through smoking or using a vaporizer pen. You'll also have to ask yourself another important question: Do I want to feel high? You might opt for a high-CBD strain like Charlotte's Web or Dancehall, or maybe you prefer something more balanced, such as a strain containing equal parts THC and CBD, like Warlock, which will bring about a lighter high than a more THC-dominant strain. Perhaps you prefer the euphoria that comes with a little more THC—some definitely do! (I once met an MMA fighter who said she enjoyed doing a few bong hits of her favorite uplifting strain before hitting the pads at practice.) Even I, barely an athlete, have experienced the benefit of a little prerun toke: to paraphrase Rebagliati, the task at hand seems simplified, and I'm able to focus on what I'm doing without stressing about the steep hill or miserable weather I'll have to face.

Post-workout, the variety of options is almost too wide to list here. Oils, tinctures, capsules, infused energy bars, tonics, waters, and just about every other edible product you can imagine exist in some facet of the market, with the greatest variety in the United States. While cannabis legalization might seem far off in certain parts of the world, products made from hemp-derived CBD are becoming more and more accepted in North America and parts of Europe, with organizations like the World Anti-Doping Agency even removing CBD from its list of banned substances in 2017. I tend to agree with Rebagliati—it's more than plausible that CBD-infused products will soon be sold in grocery stores like Whole Foods, between aisles of supplements and protein powder.

Two options for consuming cannabis are inhalation or ingestion, but if you're still uncomfortable with the idea of either of these, consider a topical. While I'm sure remedies like Tiger Balm will never lose their place in the world, THC-infused creams, balms, salves, and patches are a great way to experience the benefits of this powerful compound without experiencing the intoxicating effects that come with consuming THC. (Just be sure not to ingest any of it or let your children or pets get at it.)

CANNABIS AS A SUPERFOOD

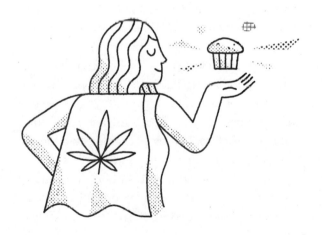

Case Study: Mary Jean "Watermelon" Dunsdon
....

A WOMAN OF legendary status in Canada's cannabis industry, Mary Jean "Watermelon" Dunsdon has
been cooking and baking with cannabis since 1993.

"The year you were born!" she jokes as we speak
over the phone. (I tell her I'm a little older than that,
but she's not far off.) Known in B.C. and beyond
for being arrested in 2001 at Vancouver's clothing-
optional beach for selling her famously delicious
"special" ginger snaps, she's come a long way from
her days of slinging *actual* slices of watermelon
and infused goodies, and now operates two specialty candy stores in the city. (No, the candy is not
infused.)

"I've always been obsessed with baking and
cooking—since I was a child," she says. "Back then,
you heard about brownies the odd person made

every once in a while, but there were no retailers around. I found a need and filled it with two of my favorite things: weed and food."

She's since retired from her unofficial job at the beach, but she remains both a strong proponent of combining food and marijuana and an advocate for the plant and the people who use it. As a decades-long user, Watermelon credits the good herb with many things, but especially with keeping her young and healthy. And at forty-five, let me tell you, Watermelon looks pretty damn good for her age.

"Absolutely, 100 percent," she says when I ask if the herb has anything to do with it. "Cannabis has kept me young and sexy—it's absolutely the fountain of youth. It's the greatest thing for women as they age."

While she's always enjoyed consuming cannabis recreationally, she's noticed that as she's gotten older, her use has unintentionally become more therapeutic in nature. A THC capsule she once enjoyed taking a few nights a week to "chill out" before bed has become a more regular occurrence since she realized how much it helped her sleep and eased her pain and hormonal imbalances.

Beyond consuming it in capsules or one of her famous infused meals, Watermelon enjoys eating cannabis in every way possible—from options like putting hemp seeds on her yogurt to juicing raw cannabis and fan leaves into ice cube trays for future use in shakes, smoothies, and even plain old water. In her opinion, the nutrient-rich plant should be lumped in with vegetables instead of narcotics. (Raw cannabis, like hemp, is not intoxicating—it's heat that converts the nonintoxicating tetrahydrocannabinolic acid (THCA) found in raw plants to the psychoactive THC.)

"Cannabis is a green leafy vegetable. Your mother told you to eat your greens. She meant cannabis— she just didn't know it at the time," she says. "It's packed with a lot of different nutrients, so it's a 'superfood' in that way—it's a green, like kale and spinach. I always go back to the idea that just because somebody decided to separate this green leafy vegetable from the team, somehow we've vilified it, and we think about it differently, instead of looking at it for what it really is."

What Makes a "Superfood"?

ACAI BERRIES, ALMONDS, asparagus, avocados... and that barely covers the a's: North America's ongoing obsession with "superfoods"—nutrient-dense foods that support numerous functions of the body and are considered by nutritionists to be highly beneficial for health and well-being—may be annoying, but it's a long overdue trend for a continent plagued with obesity and disease. Given what we've already learned about cannabis in this book—that it's high in medicinal compounds that can help us sleep, decrease stress, lift our moods, and keep us slim—who's to say it can't be included in the superfoods group? A 2018 story (published on April 20, no less) in the *Washington Post* confirmed my suspicion that this idea has already been introduced to the mainstream. In "Milk, Bread, Hemp Oil? A Dietitian's Guide to the Cannabis Items in Your Grocery Store," Christy Brissette says certain cannabis-derived products are already widely available in the U.S., despite marijuana's being illegal at the federal level.

"Cannabis is making its way into more and more foods and beverages, thanks to its touted therapeutic benefits. In fact, no matter where you are in the United States, cannabis products are probably being sold in your grocery store—and it's perfectly legal,"[1] she writes, before explaining the differences between hemp (a variety of cannabis bred for fiber and edible seeds) and "marijuana" (the type of cannabis we've been talking about up until this point, bred for its medical and recreational uses). Both hemp seeds and their oil are high in omega-3 and omega-6 fatty acids, with the seeds containing over 30 percent healthy fat and more than 25 percent protein—significantly more than flax or chia seeds—as well as vitamin E and minerals like phosphorus, sodium, potassium, sulfur, magnesium, zinc, calcium, and iron.

Hemp seeds and oil are certainly more accessible options when it comes to both availability and cost; plus, they also allow consumers to experience the benefits of "cannabis" without the intoxication that comes with consuming a variety of the plant that makes you high. On top of that, hemp can be used to create milk, flour, protein powder, cereal, and snacks—and that's just food. An incredibly durable material, hemp can be used for both fiber and fuel (hell, even Rudolf Diesel invented the world's first diesel engine with the intention of running it on vegetable oils like hemp oil) and has been used in tens of thousands of products, including as the material used to build the bodies of cars, trucks, and even airplanes.

That being said, there is growing interest in how ingesting various parts of the cannabis plant in its raw form—from roots to seeds to leaves—can provide similar benefits to those of the superfoods mentioned earlier in this chapter.

History of Cannabis as a Superfood

IT IS WIDELY believed that hemp was one of the first plants cultivated by humans for textiles and fiber as far back as twelve thousand years ago— older readers might recall Carl Sagan's suggestion in 1977 that hemp may have been the world's first crop, thereby leading to civilization as we know it—so is it a stretch to assume that it was also being used as a source of food?

While records of exactly how it was consumed in certain areas are more difficult to find, one record of hemp as food comes from a story that has been passed around cannabis-user circles since it was written in *The Emperor Wears No Clothes*, the widely published book by the Emperor of Hemp, Jack Herer: "Many Buddhist traditions, writings, and beliefs indicate that 'Siddhartha' [the Buddha] himself, used and ate nothing but hemp and its seeds for six years prior to announcing [discovering] his truths and becoming the Buddha."[2] I'll leave it to those on Internet Buddhism forums to debate whether or not this story is in fact based on truth—it's really just one example of the use of hemp for food—but, even if the Buddha himself didn't eat hemp or its derivatives, it's estimated that cannabis seeds and oil were being used for food as early as 6000 BCE. Interestingly, the *Shennong Ben Cao Jing*, dated to 2737 BCE, notes the use of hemp roots as pain medicine. (The point man on cannabis roots, Dr. Ethan Russo, told me that while the contents of the plant's roots are pharmacologically very different from cannabis flowers, they were historically used to treat the same kinds of problems, including pain and inflammation.) We know it was also used in India, in a drinkable preparation that combined *bhang*, a cannabis paste, with milk, ghee, and spices, in around 2000 BCE.

While the use of hemp eventually spread from modern-day Asia to northern Europe in 500 BCE, indications that it was used in the region as fiber are much stronger than indications that it was used as food, until around medieval times, when it was used as an alternative to flax. Then, in the fifteenth century, an Italian scholar by the name of Bartolomeo Platina published a cookbook in Latin called *De honesta voluptate* (On honest pleasure). In it were several recipes that called for cannabis, including one called *cibarium cannabinum*,[3] or cannabis soup: "Make a hemp dish for twelve guests this way: cook a pound of well-washed hemp until it splits open. When it is cooked, add a pound of almonds. When it has been pounded with bread crumbs in a mortar, moisten it with lean stock.... When it is almost cooked, put in a half pound of sugar, a half ounce of ginger, and a little saffron with rose water."[4]

Eventually imported into North America, hemp was a popular industry until the 1930s. But when bankers with investments in the oil, paper, synthetic fiber, plastic, and pharmaceuticals industries felt threatened by the technological advancements being made with hemp, they called on newly appointed commissioner of the Federal Bureau of Narcotics Harry Anslinger and launched a campaign that would eventually scare the public into believing that hemp was bad, and worse, that cannabis would cause African Americans and Mexicans to commit crimes against white women and children.

While hemp products marketed as superfoods are once again widely available, the impact of Anslinger's war on hemp and cannabis cannot be overlooked. Its implications for fiber and fuel alone are enough to leave me speechless, but that's for another book. Thankfully, the demonization of a plant with enormous therapeutic potential seems to be coming to an end, as cannabis slowly sheds its reputation as a dirty weed and blooms into a powerful superfood.

How Cannabis Can Help

WHEN ROBYN GRIGGS Lawrence received her medical marijuana card from her gynecologist in 2009, it was a revelation of sorts for the full-time magazine editor, health-focused foodie, volleyball mom, and self-proclaimed "research chef," who still felt skeptical on her first trip to a local medical cannabis dispensary.

Instead of visiting a shop in her neighborhood—"at this point there was one on every block"—Lawrence says she drove to a dispensary in the next town for fear of running into other volleyball parents. Recalling her encounter with medical cannabis on that initial trip, Lawrence says she was blown away by the range of products available at her fingertips.

"I had no idea that cannabis came in 'flavors,'" she says, referencing the numerous different strains or cultivars on display in the dispensary. "The last I'd seen of it was back in the eighties, when it was sticks and seeds and didn't really smell like anything." The idea that different types of cannabis had different smells, colors, textures, and tasting notes wasn't something she had considered.

In that moment, Lawrence knew that what she had come across was far more than just an herb to be smoked. "When the budtender pulled it down for me and let me smell it, I thought, wow, this is incredible—Lemon Skunk actually does smell like lemon, and Chocolope actually smells like chocolate!"

"Oh my God," she thought to herself. "This is food." Being a mom who had instilled healthy values into her children, Lawrence didn't want to smoke, so she knew that edibles would be her preferred method of consumption. But at the time, most edible products on the market were packed with sugar—a vice she prefers to avoid. Rather than opting for high-priced infused sweets, Lawrence took it upon herself to learn the ins and outs of cooking with cannabis and using it in her food. As a journalist, this was definitely in her wheelhouse, but she tells me she never imagined that it would lead to writing a book of her own—*The Cannabis Kitchen Cookbook*—a collaborative project that involved consulting with some of the world's top "cannabis chefs."

"I live in Boulder, Colorado, and everyone has a special diet here," she says with a laugh. Between the vegans, vegetarians, gluten and dairy abstainers, and Paleo dieters, Lawrence says dietary restrictions make it difficult to host a dinner party—never mind an infused one. But by teaming up with chefs who shared her interest in specialty foods and organic ingredients, she was able to create a unique cookbook that not only provided cannabis users with health-conscious infused recipes, but also demystified the plant that had positively affected the lives of the chefs she worked with. "Pretty much every chef in that cookbook had someone in their lives that cannabis had made a difference for," she says. "They just wanted to get this out there, to empower people to be able to do it themselves, and to me, out of all the projects I've ever done, that was the most amazing thing."

Having developed hundreds of recipes over the years, incorporating both cannabis that has been decarboxylated—a chemical change that transforms the precursor THCA into the psychoactive compound THC—and different parts of the plant in its raw form, Lawrence has become intensely familiar with the plant's nutritious components. "One thing that people don't realize is that cannabis is actually classified as a vegetable," she says. "It's full of antioxidants, magnesium, zinc, and vitamins, and really is a fantastic nutritional food in its raw form. When you're pulling cannabinoids out to cook to make an oil or an extraction, you're getting the benefits of those cannabinoids and terpenes, but the best way to get the full nutritional profile and benefits is to eat it raw." An added benefit? Because the chemical change that activates THC hasn't occurred, fresh, raw cannabis won't get you high, though Lawrence does warn that she's been challenged on that fact by an ethnobotanist or two. While most agree that consuming raw cannabis won't lead to feelings of intoxication,[5] cannabis that has been dried or cured will have already begun the process of decarboxylation, albeit rather slowly, so it's best to use fresh cannabis if you want to avoid feeling high.

Unfortunately, she says, despite the fact that raw cannabis plants aren't intoxicating, society seems to have lumped them in with the stuff that makes you "high." A perfect example of this is the way certain parts of the cannabis plant are considered "waste," even in her cannabis-friendly home state of Colorado. "It's too bad, because the fan leaves are such a wonderful, beautiful nutritional piece, and they just get composted or thrown away. Here in Colorado, you can't get them from growers, because everything is regulated, even their garbage." Lawrence likens it to "throwing away tons of spectacular food every day," and says the lack of understanding is very frustrating.

In time, she hopes more people will catch on to the notion that cannabis is indeed a superfood—but she says it's worth trying to push that classification a step further. "'Superfood' is unfortunately a word that has gotten so overused, but if we look at the contemporary definition of the way we're using it, cannabis is definitely a superfood."

A couple of quick facts about the plant we've come to know and, for the most part, smoke: while we can obtain some cannabinoids through inhalation, cannabinoids are fat-soluble, and ingesting them allows us to absorb them better. Perhaps one of the best-known proponents of the raw cannabis movement is U.S. doctor and cannabis researcher Dr. William Courtney. He calls raw cannabis "a dietary essential," and swears by its therapeutic effects on patients. Not only is raw cannabis high in fiber, polyphenols, flavonoids, amino acids, essential oils, and minerals like magnesium, calcium, and phosphorus, it's also higher in cannabinoids. Courtney has said that raw cannabis could be an option for everyone because it allows for greater consumption of the active cannabinoids (up to sixty times as many as when the cannabis is heated) without the risk of getting high.

Using Cannabis as a Superfood

NOW, AFTER THAT last section, you may be asking yourself the very question I found myself posing to Lawrence: This whole raw cannabis thing sounds great, but how does one acquire fresh buds and leaves?

Unfortunately (and unlike other leafy green vegetables), the parts of the plant useful for raw consumption can't be obtained at a grocery store. Unless you live in a part of the world where personal cultivation of cannabis is legal, getting your hands on trim and leaves might require making friends with a local black market grower, or, you know, breaking the law and growing a few plants in your closet. Adult residents of Colorado are allowed to grow up to six plants on their own property, and while that provision comes with a host of stipulations, Lawrence says it's a common choice among people in her hometown. If she didn't grow cannabis at home, she says, she wouldn't have access to critical ingredients like fresh buds and fan leaves.

Besides Colorado, other states that allow the home cultivation of cannabis at time of writing include Alaska, Arizona, California, District of Columbia, Hawaii, Maine, Massachusetts, Michigan,

Montana, Nevada, New Mexico, North Dakota, Oregon, Rhode Island, Vermont, and Washington, with the majority providing a license to grow to approved patients only and not recreational users. Legislation in Canada has legalized the home cultivation of cannabis for adults, allowing them to grow up to four plants per household. Canadians in all provinces and territories except Manitoba and Quebec will be able to purchase seeds and plants from licensed producers. Approved patients in Canada have, for the most part, been allowed to grow their own cannabis since 2001. Just Uruguay has completely legalized recreational use and allows its citizens to grow their own cannabis, while other countries like Spain, Mexico, and Jamaica have decriminalized cannabis and allow personal cultivation. In Australia, only licensed medical patients can grow their own cannabis.

Lawrence recognizes the importance of being able to grow her own plants: "We're incredibly fortunate that we have this option, because it's really hard to get anything other than flower from growers or a dispensary." At the time of our discussion, her freezer was full of homemade pesto made with a combination of cannabis leaves and basil. She says the leaves can also add unique flavor when included in a salad or sprinkled on a soup, while both leaves and raw buds can be easily integrated into juices, smoothies, and shakes.

She recommends using only leaves and flowers picked from an organically grown plant during its early flower stage. As with vegetables purchased in a supermarket, she recommends a thorough wash and soak to remove any dirt. Soaking also helps to soften the leaves.

While consuming raw cannabis does add a lot of valuable nutritional components to her diet, Lawrence says she has absolutely nothing against the euphoria that comes with ingesting cannabis that has been decarboxylated, and she likes to use coconut oil to create her own infused oils. "It's a really great fat to use because it really takes on the THC and CBD. It's a 'good' fat too, and really, the fattier the better when you're making this kind of extraction," she says.

If creating your own oil seems too complicated, worry not. Lawrence says decarboxylating cannabis is actually a lot easier than the average person might think. She says it can be as easy as putting your cannabis on a cookie sheet and baking it in an oven at a low temperature (180°F to 250°F depending on your oven) for about 15 minutes. *That's it?!*

"That's it," she says. "Decarboxylation is what we did when we lit a pipe—it's a super-simple process." She says she's always learning about new ways to decarboxylate cannabis. While there is much discussion—even controversy—around what the "best" way might be, she notes that every chef she spoke with for her book (over a dozen) preferred a different method of decarboxylation.

In some instances, activating the cannabis can simply be done during cooking: if you thought bacon was already too good to be true (apologies to the vegetarians and vegans reading), it can be made even more wonderful by simply sprinkling a little cannabis on top while it's in the frying pan (cook at a low temperature for best results). Remember Watermelon? One of her favorite recipes for B.C. Baked Salmon involves a similar method, with dried cannabis (preferably B.C. bud) being added to a slab of freshly caught wild salmon before being baked in the oven. And if you've got a slow cooker, Lawrence says the flavors brought out by adding cannabis to a pork roast are nothing short of amazing.

While she doesn't call herself a chef, she enjoys throwing the odd cannabis-oriented dinner party, and says one of the biggest differences between a traditional dinner and one that's been infused is alcohol. "For one thing, you'll remember it all the next day, and you won't wake up feeling miserable." Maybe you'll have accidently fallen asleep on the couch, but chances are you've had a pretty good night's rest.

For hosts, Lawrence says it's key to keep doses low—even lower than what you already think is safe—because each of your guests is going to have

a different reaction based on their tolerance, especially if their last exposure to cannabis was during
the Grateful Dead tour of '77. "People think they
want to eat an entire infused meal, but they don't,"
she says. "One of the things I've learned is that
every portion needs to be way lower [in cannabis
content] than what you expected."

Because of the way cannabinoids interact with
other ingredients in the food, Lawrence says there's
a building effect that can cause even small doses to
make a big difference to someone's level of intoxication. That's why, she says, 2.5 milligrams in a
dessert could feel like 10 if guests have been ingesting cannabinoids throughout dinner. "If you eat
too much [cannabis-infused] food, it's definitely
not like smoking too much," she says as I vigor-
ously nod in agreement. While no one has ever died
from overdosing on THC, ingesting too much of it
can lead to rapid heart rate, hallucinations, confusion, or paranoia.[6] "It's awful—you won't die, but
you might feel like you are," she jokes. Been there,
done that.

An easy way to mitigate responsibility as a chef
is to offer the infused portion of the meal as a sauce
on the side or in a salad dressing. "That way everybody controls their own destiny," Lawrence says.
Other dinner party tips include ensuring that all
parties have a safe ride home, and that tasty non-
alcoholic beverages are always available for those
who feel naked without a drink in their hand.

I'll admit I find the idea of throwing an infused dinner party terrifying—but obtaining the benefits of decarboxylated cannabis doesn't need to involve such an undertaking. It can be as easy as adding your own infused oil to your tea or coffee in the morning. (While pre-infused cooking oils can be purchased from certain manufacturers, creating your own oils with home-grown cannabis or relatively inexpensive flower from a dispensary not only gives you control, it's also a lot more affordable.)

"Once you understand the basic science of turning THCA to THC, and that it's fat-soluble, you can do anything   if you like cooking. If you don't, then this might not be for you," Lawrence says.

Her advice to novice cooks interested in giving decarboxylation a try? You might say it's the same advice you'd give to a person about to indulge in edibles. "Start small! Don't start with an ounce. Practice with a gram, because there is nothing worse than making a mistake and burning your bud," she says, speaking from experience. As for tasting, she advises that even if you have complete confidence in the strength of what you've made, there are many factors that come into play and could affect the potency of the oil.

"That's what scares people the most about this food—it's so easy to slip into 'had too much,'" she says. "The whole 'start low and go slow' thing—it's kind of our mantra in Colorado."

6
...

A STEAMIER
SEX LIFE

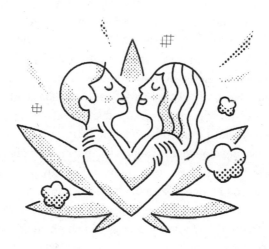

Case Study: Lisa "Mamakind" Kirkman
....

CANADIAN AUTHOR AND cannabis columnist Lisa "Mamakind" Kirkman lives in Calgary, Alberta, where she spends her days writing cannabis-related stories and answering questions from cannabis users looking to literally spice up their sex life... with weed. The forty-three-year-old has made a career out of combining cannabis and sex—Rihanna even Instagrammed her book *Sex Pot*, calling it her "new encyclopedia"—though she tells me by phone that her first foray into the world of infused play happened when she was alone. "To be honest it was a masturbatory thing," she says. "I masturbated with it for the first time after getting high, and I was like, 'Wait a minute... this is so much better!'" she says with a laugh.

In university, when cannabis seemed to be available everywhere, Kirkman says she began using it daily, and noticed that sex with her boy-friend was more enjoyable after indulging in a puff. "My explorations into sex and cannabinoids basically happened sort of naturally, as I explored my own sexuality," she recalls. From as early as she can remember and right into early adulthood, Kirkman tells me she was self-conscious about her body and sometimes had a hard time meeting people. Not only did cannabis serve her well in the bedroom, it also made the process of meeting new people and future intimate partners far less stressful.

"Before you have sex with anybody you have to meet them, talk with them, and connect on some level, other than just physically. Smoking cannabis, you're usually standing in a circle, doing something illegal, and it forces everybody together in a little group—it's a very intimate experience in and of itself," she says. Being the source of the cannabis on a night out doesn't hurt either. "When you have a joint, it draws people in, and it becomes something you can talk about. Plus, you're already sharing fluids with somebody, so there's that," she laughs.

The relaxation brought on by using cannabis also made sex happen more frequently for Lisa, who felt less insecure about her body after smoking a joint. "I became relaxed enough that my confidence started shining through," she says. That same relaxation carried over to the bedroom, nullifying her anxiety while heightening her senses and making her more emotionally open. "I noticed it opened me up and allowed me to go with the flow and enjoy myself, to really be mindful of the feelings that I was having—and not being panicked," she says.

Lisa talks about the pressure women put on themselves in the bedroom to both perform for their partners and reach orgasm. Not only does using cannabis make her feel closer to and more intimate with her partner, she says, it also makes her more aware of her partner's needs.

Being extra turned on by her partner is one thing, but Lisa admits there's something sexy about the herb itself. "I get turned on by weed, I really do—the paraphernalia, the smell of it—it just gets me going," she says, adding that for those interested in a little kink, cannabis itself can be a tool in the bedroom: "roach play" is a term she coined that involves using a joint in place of candle wax or a feather to tease your partner. But if that's too much for you, she says, there are definitely easier ways to bring cannabis into the bedroom.

Enhancing Sex and Sensuality

FROM VIBRATORS TO Viagra and penis pumps to pleasure oil, humans seem to be obsessed with increasing sexual desire, upping sexual performance, and maximizing sexual pleasure.

A STEAMIER SEX LIFE

If a prudish upbringing has led you to believe that the phenomenon of treating sex in this way is a side effect of pop culture putting too much emphasis on sex and sexuality, I've got news for you: the ancient Egyptians used aphrodisiacs, and yes, even sought ways to lengthen their penises. Sex-specific drugs—whether they were taken for the reasons listed above, or to prevent pregnancy and disease—have existed for literally ages. And while the idea of using cannabis in this way may seem strange or even unlikely, history tells us that it wasn't uncommon.

Historical Use of Cannabis for Sex

WHILE IT'S NOT exactly sex, it's certainly the result of intercourse: one of the earliest recorded sex-related uses of cannabis was for childbirth. In ancient Egypt, women applied cannabis to the inside of their vaginas to ease the pain of, well, childbirth. There are numerous records of its being used for this throughout history, and while the Egyptians applied extractions or oils, others used cannabis smoke, burning it and then administering it to women in labor.[1] Its use as an aphrodisiac was also common.

Cannabis was also used in conjunction with sex in India in about 700 CE. Its use for both tantric sex and yoga arose out of what researcher Dr. Michael

Aldrich calls "an explosive mingling" of different elements of Shaivite Hinduism and Tibetan Buddhism. "The tradition of drug yoga is an ancient and honorable one in India, developed to its fullest extent in tantric practice," he writes. "The Tantras transform Hindu sexual practices into a means of meditational yoga. Marijuana fits into sex yoga as well, for in Hindu folk medicine it is the aphrodisiac *par excellence*."[2] Cannabis served not as a "disinhibiting agent," but as an awareness booster that was essential to tantric ceremonies.

It is believed that the Vikings who worshipped the Norse goddess Freya also indulged in cannabis as an aphrodisiac. Freya, considered the goddess of love, was associated with hemp, so at sowing and harvesting times each year, cannabis flowers were consumed and erotic rituals were held in her name.[3]

In his observations of the effects of cannabis, Irish physician William O'Shaughnessy wrote in 1843 that one preparation was "most fascinating in its effects, producing ecstatic happiness, a persuasion of high rank, a sensation of flying, voracious appetite, and intense aphrodisiac desire."[4]

In more recent history, a 1975 paper by anthropologist Sula Benet shows that cannabis was used in Soviet Russia in the 1930s both as an aphrodisiac and for pain relief. Cannabis was mixed with lamb's fat to create a mixture called *nasha*, which was given to brides in the evening of their wedding day to reduce the pain of first intercourse. Candy containing hashish, called *guc-kand*, was made for boys who were suffering from pain caused by circumcision. Women would sometimes add tobacco to another *nasha*-like substance and apply it to the inside of their vaginas to make them tighter. Don't worry, guys, women didn't get to have all the fun— men often indulged in what they called "happy porridge," an aphrodisiacal combination of hemp flowers, seeds, and spices.[5]

While cannabis is illegal in Uganda, traditional healers have used it to help men suffering from erectile dysfunction for many years. According to a study published in 2005, cannabis is one of numerous plants used by healers to manage sexual impotence.[6] It is typically smoked.

In my opinion, no discussion of the intersection of cannabis and sex would be complete without at least mentioning the year 1967. The Summer of Love and the years that followed gave birth to a new way of thinking about sex, drugs, and life in general that have come to shape some of our current discourse around both sexual identity and drug use. I simply can't ignore the fact that cannabis had a massive presence at the Be-Ins, Smoke-Ins, festivals, and "beatnik gatherings" where the youths of yesteryear gathered together in the interest of "free love." (It's ironic that many of the people who grew up in the sixties are now completely anti-pot. Go figure.)

How Cannabis Can Help
....

CLEARLY, IT'S NOT hard to find historical and anecdotal cases of cannabis being used not just to facilitate sex, but also to make it more enjoyable. As with many subjects in this book, much of the initial research that has been conducted by scientists was done with the hopes of uncovering something negative—and the same can be said for the research into cannabis and sex. While scientists have certainly tried to link cannabis use to things like sexual dysfunction and "high-risk" behavior or promiscuity, there is also evidence to show that cannabis can not only increase sexual pleasure and satisfaction, it may also increase desire.

In the 1970s and particularly in the 1980s, researchers took a keen interest in cannabis and sex. An early study by Dr. Wayne C. Koff in 1974 found that cannabis led to increased sexual motivation.[7] Another, by Ronald A. Weller and James A. Halikas and published in *The Journal of Sex Research* in 1984, attempted to determine the perceived effects of cannabis on sexual behavior and practices by interviewing groups of cannabis users and non-users. It found that over two-thirds of subjects reported increased sexual pleasure and satisfaction when using cannabis, while about half reported feeling increased sexual desire for a familiar sexual partner. About half told the researchers conducting the study that they viewed cannabis as an aphro-disiac and felt enhanced senses of touch and taste, while about 20 percent of the subjects said they used cannabis before sex regularly.[8]

After that, research on the topic seemed to fall off for about twenty years. Similar survey-type studies were conducted by two different groups of Canadian researchers in 2003 and 2008, with both coming to similar conclusions as the U.S. survey conducted in 1984, but little research has looked at the more specific implications of exactly *how* cannabinoids serve us in the bedroom. In fact, one study conducted in 2015 actually looked into whether or not cannabis use decreased men's sperm count. By comparing samples from users and nonusers, the study found that men who smoked cannabis regularly had 29 percent lower sperm count than their counterparts who abstained. When combined with other recreational drug use, sperm count was lowered even further, by 55 percent.[9]

The research landscape changed with the pub-lication of a study in the journal *Current Sexual Health Reports* in 2017. Researcher Dr. Richard Balon of Wayne State University found that can-nabis actually has a bidirectional effect on sexual functioning: at low doses, it may promote sexual arousal and enhance functioning, but at higher doses, not only will sex be less enjoyable, but regular use may lead to negative effects, including lack of interest, erectile dysfunction, and inhibited orgasm.[10]

Another recent study asked an entirely different question: Do cannabis users have more sex than nonusers? Based on what we've already learned about sex and cannabis in this chapter, the results probably won't surprise you. By analyzing nine years of data from nearly fifty thousand adults who responded to the annual National Survey of Family Growth, researchers found that across all demographics, women who used cannabis either monthly, weekly, or daily had significantly higher sexual frequency than those who did not use cannabis. Men who consumed cannabis either weekly or daily had similar results. While the study stated that consumption did not appear to impair sexual function, it also called for further research on the relationship between sex and cannabis.[11]

Given the nature of the research on this topic and the consensus among cannabis users that the plant is indeed a great tool for better sex, speaking with a sex educator rather than an academic seemed appropriate.

An author, workshop facilitator, and pleasure and communications coach, Ashley Manta is the cannabis industry's answer to Dr. Ruth Westheimer. The California native coined (and federally trademarked) the term "CannaSexual," and while she says some confuse it with a sexual orientation, it's meant to describe anyone who mindfully and deliberately combines sex and cannabis.

"It's really meant to be a word that's not only a brand but a philosophy, an approach, a mind-set," she tells me by phone. The inclusive, sex-positive workshops she teaches cover topics like "All Hands on Bits! Hand Sex for All Bodies," "Sexy Supplies: An Intro to Toys, Lube, and Accessories," and of course, "Light My Fire: How Cannabis Can Enhance Pleasure."

"They come from a place of 'Let's throw out everything you think you know about cannabis, or how to use cannabis, or even how to have sex,'" she says. "I like to give [attendees] a new paradigm to work with that focuses on pleasure, consent, embodiment, presence, and mindfulness."

In her mind, the benefits of combining sex and cannabis are infinite, and can manifest in many different ways. People who deal with chronic pain, she says, might struggle with intimacy because their pain distracts them from being present with their partner. Cannabis can not only help quiet the pain, but also help keep them in the right state of mind. The same could go for people who struggle with stress and anxiety.

"Regardless of what kind of equipment you're working with, whether you have a vulva or a penis, we all struggle with similar things when it comes to arousal and body confidence," she says. "Like the things that we believe about the way that our bodies are supposed to interact with each other, or what sex is supposed to look like. Cannabis helps you break out of that mold."

Opening up about her own reason for using cannabis in the bedroom, Manta says her first foray into using cannabis for sex was with an infused topical. "The reason I stumbled onto cannabis for sex was because I have pain with penetration from a history of sexual trauma," she says. "Using cannabis topically was the first time I was ever able to have penetrative sex without pain." Pain with penetrative sex is common among people with vulvas, she says, for a variety of reasons.

Menopause is another life event that Manta says can be positively affected by cannabis use. "Cisgender women specifically might suffer from vaginal dryness, atrophy, and pain, just because of the way the tissue changes," she says, noting that some women have also used cannabis as a supplement to hormone replacement therapy to help deal with hot flashes and other symptoms of menopause. Women with endometriosis could also benefit from cannabis use, she says.

"But cannabis can also be used as an enhancer, not just addressing the things that are getting in the way of connection and pleasure," she says, "but also enhancing pleasurable sensations and sensory perception, because THC and CBD, to a lesser extent, do help to bring your body online."

Using Cannabis for Sex

WITH SO MANY reasons to try integrating cannabis into your sex life, I bet you're wondering what the first step might be: Is it smoking or vaporizing? Is it using a topical? Is it happy porridge? (I digress.)

"One of the first things I always like to let people know is that you don't have to have psychoactive effects to enjoy the benefits of cannabis and sex," says Manta. There are plenty of ways to use cannabis that don't require getting high but can still enhance your sexual experience. Using an infused topical, like a pleasure oil, she says, is a great place to begin. And of course, she notes that it doesn't necessarily require a partner.

"A topical can be a really useful tool to have in your arsenal so that you can connect with your partner more deeply, or connect with yourself," she says. A high-CBD strain is another option for people who might be dealing with pre-sex nerves and don't want to feel high.

Manta says it's especially important for couples to ask themselves what kind of sex they want to be having.

"If you're going for slow, lovemaking sex, I'm definitely going to give a different recommendation than if you're looking for frenzied, lustful, pounding sex," she says. She also considers significant factors like time, finances, tolerance, and past experiences with cannabis when she's consulting with a couple for the first time. Once the "intake" process is complete, she starts suggesting specific products and methods of ingestion that are suitable for what they're looking for.

Manta says she's developed her own little collection of favorite strains for sex and that keeping track of what works for you is a vital tool for integrating cannabis and sex. "I like to get people to look at cannabinoid and terpene profiles, because then they know their cannabis is being tested," she says. For the most part, she tries to strike a balance when making recommendations, because she doesn't want clients to be disappointed if a certain product doesn't work. "Find what works for you and your body and make the medicine work for you—don't try to force yourself into a mold that doesn't fit," she says.

In Manta's own sex life, her goal is always "to make sex as connected, passionate, pleasurable, and fun in each moment." It's why she prefers to use strains that are a bit more playful and euphoric, in conjunction with other tools, like topicals and toys. "When my boyfriend arrives, maybe I'll have a bowl packed with something like Lemon Larry OG, a balanced but euphoric strain high in a terpene called limonene," she says. Limonene is essentially the compound in citrus fruits (and cannabis) that gives them their distinct lemony smell. Manta says it wakes up her senses while also making her body more receptive to touch. After "shotgunning" a few hits together—shotgunning is blowing cannabis smoke directly into another person's mouth, a process that is far sexier than it sounds—kissing is unavoidable. Once her clothes are off, she'll spray a topical on her vulva and wait twenty minutes for the cannabinoids to start bringing increased blood flow to the area before getting down and dirty.

Manta likes to keep her pre-sex strains below 15 percent THC to avoid the anxiety brought on by the biphasic effects of cannabis that could cause her to get too high—a surefire way to put an abrupt end to any sexual encounter. There's a threshold to "This feels good," she says, that can quickly devolve into "I regret all of my life choices."

A good way to avoid getting too high before getting intimate, she says, is to use cannabis in conjunction with masturbation before introducing it to a partnered situation. "It's such an important self-care tool and ritual for connecting with your body, as well as an important way to create data about what cannabis does to your body sexually," she says. "If you have a new strain or a new edible or a topical product, use it however it's intended, and masturbate! Then take notes in a journal: 'This made me really turned on,' 'This really helped me get out of my head,' 'I had four orgasms'; *or*, 'I was really distracted and all I wanted to do was sleep,' 'I just got hungry and didn't feel like doing anything else.' Whatever it is, it's good data to have."

One thing to remember when using any oil-based lubricant, however, is that it can't be used with latex condoms, because it will damage them. If you intend to try one out, be sure to pick up a box of condoms made out of polyurethane or nitrile.

AN EFFECTIVE
SOURCE OF PAIN
MANAGEMENT

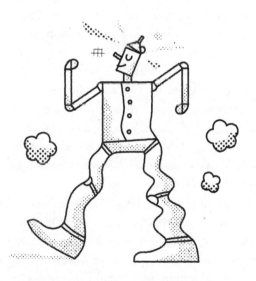

Case Study: Galen Pallas

EFFECTIVE PAIN MANAGEMENT is essential for Oakland, California, native Galen Pallas. As the founder and CEO of his own cannabis company, Kind Culture, he can't afford to have his days interrupted constantly with chronic pain—pain that is often intensified by violent twitches. Pallas was diagnosed with Tourette's syndrome as a preteen, and says while it's often characterized by vocal and physical tics, he suffers from "twitches, not swears." When I ask what causes his chronic pain, he tells me there isn't one simple answer.

"It's complex," he says. "My body makes jerky movements in my head, neck, and shoulders that I cannot control." These jerky movements cause intense headaches and, after years of the same repetitive motion, severe pain in the back, neck, and shoulders. Following his diagnosis, he says, he was put on so many different medications that he felt like a guinea pig. When he began smoking cannabis recreationally as a teenager, it did something for him that other drugs could not: not only did it reduce the number of headaches he experienced, it also limited the frequency and severity of his twitches.

The year he graduated from high school, the state of California legalized medical cannabis, and at age eighteen, Pallas was among the first one thousand Americans to receive a prescription. Though it served him well in college, he says he stopped using it once he began working and no longer enjoyed the feeling of being high.

When he began experiencing intense chronic pain several years later, his doctor's first line of defense was opioids. He says they worked incredibly well for a few years, but when his pain eventually became so intense that his doctor could no longer increase his dose, surgery was the only remaining option.

Describing the brutal surgery, Pallas says it was like having his cervical spine cut in half and then put back together. Doctors instructed him not to move his neck for three months after the procedure, but his twitches made keeping still next to impossible. When the pain medication he was being given didn't adequately manage the added discomfort brought on by his Tourette's, Pallas reintroduced himself to cannabis and found a combination of cannabinoids that managed his pain without making him feel impaired.

"To be honest, I can't stand the feeling of being high," he admits. "It's great recreationally, but imagine trying to run a company stoned. I know a lot of people who are capable of doing it, and God bless them, but I just don't have that skill set."

While a hemp-based CBD extract containing no THC worked to mask his physical pain, he says, "there [was] still the acute awareness that I constantly hurt." After introducing a small amount of THC in a 10:1 CBD-to-THC edible, he noticed that he was able to keep his mind calm while experiencing intense pain. "If my [baseline pain] gets exacerbated by any number of things—if I overexert myself, if I don't get a good night's sleep, if I lift something too heavy—I go into a pain cycle where it becomes almost unmanageable with medication," he says. "But the THC does a really good job of allowing my brain to focus on something besides the fact that I hurt so bad, I want to effing die." To manage chronic pain, he takes a regular dose of the edible, and when breakthrough pain hits, he sometimes supplements with a vaporizer loaded with a 95 percent CBD concentrate.

Other medications may have had a stronger effect on his physical pain, he says, but they affect other areas of his life in a negative way—things that don't seem to be affected by his cannabis use at all. "My overall energy level, my desire to communicate, talk, my sexual drive, all of those things are decreased to a noticeable level. But with cannabis, I'm able to not worry about those things, and be myself."

Pain: Why It Occurs and How We Experience It

IN MY EXPERIENCE, humans don't seem to agree on much, but I think it's fair to say we can all agree that being in a prolonged state of physical pain is not fun. Aside from generating an unpleasant feeling in the body, pain also affects our mental state, and how we perceive things: I once stubbed my toe so badly at 8 a.m.—I'm talking broken toenail, the whole nine yards—that by 4 p.m. that same day I was still fuming and ruminating on why my roommate had left his steel-toed boot in my path to the bathroom that morning.

Funny as this may be, it is not to be compared to the severity of the pain experienced by the millions—100 million in the United States alone,[1] and at least 1.5 billion people around the world[2]—who suffer from *chronic* pain. Characterized as a persistent pain that lasts longer than twelve weeks, chronic pain is the leading cause of long-term disability in the United States.[3] It affects quality of life and overall well-being in a massively profound way, with one study showing that 77 percent of people who suffered from it felt depressed because of it,[4] and another showing that more than two-thirds of the study participants said being in constant pain disrupted their sleep.[5]

Chronic pain is often neuropathic, meaning it is caused by damage to or disease of the body's somatosensory nervous system (the part of the nervous system that senses your environment), but it can also be nociceptive, or caused by damage to tissue. While patients describe the former as a shooting or burning pain, the latter tends to feel more like aching or throbbing, and is often part of the body's inflammation response to infection, wounds, or tissue damage.

Time-limited pain is often nociceptive—like the pain of stubbing my toe, or the pain you might experience after pulling a muscle or twisting your ankle. For short-term pain, it's common for us to lean on over-the-counter medications like acetaminophen (Tylenol) or ibuprofen (Advil) to help reduce the pain. While these drugs certainly have their place in treating pain, overuse can lead to toxic hepatitis, ulcers, internal bleeding, and other adverse effects. More severe nociceptive pain might be treated with an opioid, an equally important type of drug in our pharmacopeia, but one that, when overprescribed and unmanaged, can have dire consequences. Pharmaceutical drugs have certainly become the standard of care, and while it might seem as though cannabis is just emerging as a natural pain reliever, the truth is it's been used to help manage pain for more than five thousand years.

Historical Use of Cannabis for Pain

AUTHOR UWE BLESCHING writes in his 2015 book, *The Cannabis Health Index*, that cannabis was used as a pain medication in every ancient culture, including Sumer, China, Babylonia, the Indus Valley, and the Judean, Greek, Roman, and Islamic civilizations.[6] In a paper on pain management, Dr. Ethan Russo and Dr. Andrea G. Hohmann write that cannabis has been used "in one way or another for longer than written history."[7]

We learned in the last chapter that ancient Egyptians used cannabis to ease the pain of childbirth. A report commissioned by Richard Nixon in 1972 (surely intended to point out the ills of the drug and not the benefits) found that in 200 BCE, cannabis was used to quell the pain of earaches. Shen Nung recommended cannabis for more than a hundred ailments in around 1 CE, but by the second century CE, the Chinese had become so good at using cannabis that it was being combined with wine and used as an anesthetic.[8] (Funnily enough, the Chinese word for anesthesia, *mázuì*, literally translates to "cannabis intoxication.")

Pliny the Elder wrote that boiling the roots of cannabis plants in water "ease cramped joints, gout too and similar violent pain."[9] British herbalist Nicholas Culpeper wrote of using hemp to treat gout too, as well as "knots in the joints, the pains of the sinews and hips."[10] When Napoleon brought cannabis back to France in 1799, doctors were able to study both its pain-relieving and its sedative effects. It wasn't long before other parts of the Western world began to use cannabis as a remedy for pain, with Dr. William O'Shaughnessy using it to treat cramps and spasms.[11] (Even Queen Victoria used it when she suffered from monthly menstrual pain.) And the Indian Hemp Drugs Commission of 1894 (mentioned in Chapter 1) outright labeled cannabis a pain reliever.

Up until 1915, cannabis tinctures and extracts were sold in pharmacies; from 1906, they had been labeled as medicine when President Roosevelt signed the *Pure Food and Drug Act*. (If you can't picture what a nineteenth-century cannabis tincture looks like, google "Piso's Cure.") After Woodrow Wilson signed the *Harrison Narcotics Tax Act*, which would eventually be used as a model for drug regulation, in 1915, prohibition laws were enacted in ten states within the span of twelve years. Cannabis extracts remained a popular analgesic in some parts of the United States until the 1930s, when cannabis was essentially regulated into prohibition in 1937 by the Federal Bureau of Narcotics with the enactment of the *Marihuana Tax Act.*

Despite the fact that the act was opposed by the American Medical Association, doctors stopped prescribing cannabis and other drugs took its place. By 1970, cannabis was considered by U.S. Congress to be a drug with "no accepted medical use." As *if.*

How Cannabis Can Help

THE QUESTION OF whether or not cannabis can be a useful tool for pain management is not up for debate: thousands of years of its use as an analgesic combined with hundreds of patient self-report surveys generated over the last several decades tell us that people who use cannabis experience relief from pain, whether neuropathic or nociceptive. While historical use has pointed us to cannabis for pain relief, scientists are still working to understand precisely how cannabis works in this context so that it can be used more effectively. Thankfully, a greater acceptance of the plant as an analgesic in recent years has led to better quality research on the subject of exactly what cannabis, and more specifically cannabinoids, do in the body to help quell pain.

In a 2017 clinical review published in the journal *Cannabis and Cannabinoid Research*, the authors confirm that multiple randomized, controlled clinical trials show that cannabis can be an "effective pharmacotherapy for pain."[12] In examining the existing literature, it indicated that, when compared to a placebo, "cannabinoids were associated with a greater reduction in pain and greater average reduction in numerical pain ratings."

"There is converging evidence to support the notion that cannabis can produce acute pain-inhibitory effects among individuals with chronic pain," it reads.[13]

The body's endocannabinoid system plays an important role in the management of pain and inflammation. While the body's natural endocannabinoids are produced on an on-demand basis in injured tissues to help reduce pain by activating our cannabinoid receptors, cannabinoids like THC and CBD can have a similar effect on our pain tolerance. In their literature review mentioned earlier in this chapter, Russo and Hohmann write that THC is a partial agonist of both CB1 and CB2 receptors, meaning it acts as an "activator," initiating a physical response. They write that "pathological pain states have been postulated to arise, at least in part, from a dysregulation of the endocannabinoid system,"[14] meaning that an unbalanced ECS might be at least partly to blame for ongoing pain. From their examination of more than two hundred pieces of literature, they concluded that basic science and clinical trials support the idea that cannabinoid therapy is a practical way to treat chronic pain.

While we know that cannabinoids like THC and CBD can help us deal with different types of pain, scientists have (mostly) concluded that what makes cannabinoids effective is not necessarily how they interact with the pain itself, but how they interact with our perception of the pain we're experiencing. Few researchers with a focus on cannabinoid therapy have a better grasp of cannabis and its effects on pain than Dr. Mark Ware, an associate professor in family medicine and anesthesia at McGill University in Montreal, and the director of clinical research at the Alan Edwards Pain Management Unit at the McGill University Health Centre.

"Pain is a fascinating symptom," he says when I ask about how cannabis changes our perception of pain. "If you think about a pain you may have experienced, you'll know well that there's a sensory component to it, a feeling of shock from the intensity of the pain—but there's also an emotional aspect to pain," he says, describing the subsequent "I'm such an idiot" moment after you've cut yourself while cooking. "As simplistic as it sounds, it's representative of the amazing network in the brain that actually processes pain." Ware says pain signals are sent up the spinal cord and then relayed to a part of the brain called the thalamus. From there, the thalamus sends the signal throughout the brain to areas including the sensory cortex, where you feel not only the feeling of pain, but also the place in your body where the pain resides.

"It also sends out messages to the emotional centers of pain, and that starts to involve things like memory—say you've [injured yourself in this way] before—now you're even *more* of an idiot," he says, describing the way negative emotional responses like frustration, fear, and self-deprecation can affect the way we perceive pain. These reactions, he says, are all happening within split seconds of our being exposed to pain. "It may not be as obvious in an acute pain setting, when it's obvious what you've done to cause the pain, but in someone who is living with chronic pain on a daily basis, these emotional and sensory-affective components of pain are very, very important."

Ware says a cannabinoid-based drug will affect multiple centers of the brain, including memory and cognition, as well as sensation and so on. When he speaks to patients who use cannabis to treat their pain, they'll often say that while they can sometimes still feel that it's there, it doesn't come attached with the unpleasant feelings or negative emotions that it was previously associated with.

"I've heard this too many times for it just to be random: people say that it takes them away from the pain—it doesn't take the pain away from them." Explaining further, Ware describes brain-imaging studies of people suffering from experimental pain, or pain induced in a laboratory setting for the purposes of a clinical study, often used in drug development. When subjects were given THC, researchers were able to show that the part of the brain responsible for "coding the pain" as an unpleasant feeling was the amygdala. "THC binds to the receptors in the amygdala, and we think that's the reason why people report this dissociation of the pain as being painful but not unpleasant."

When I bring up the entourage effect—the idea that THC and CBD work better when offered in tandem with other cannabinoids and terpenes—Ware reminds me that, while certainly a popular one, the entourage effect is "still a bit of a hypothesis ... that all these cannabinoids and terpenes are all somehow acting in concert to create an effect that any one single agent cannot do by itself." It's certainly an attractive theory, and it might explain why whole-plant extracts of cannabis act differently than products made with single compounds.

"THC by itself does have a multitude of different effects including on pain, anxiety, appetite, muscle control—so even one compound has a multitude of different effects," he says. CBD also has myriad different characteristics, as an anti-inflammatory, an anticonvulsant, and analgesic (among others). Though scientists know less about how CBD interacts with pain than how THC does, Ware says that combining the two and then possibly adding other compounds creates more of a "wide-ranging target" than any medicine derived from a single cannabinoid ever could. In Ware's eyes, striving to understand exactly how each individual cannabinoid affects parts of the brain and body is a lofty pursuit, and one we must accept will be difficult to achieve. "You really are dealing with an incredibly complex botanical mixture. Trying to work through just what part of that symphony is working on what may actually be impossible to determine," he says. "We have to somehow embrace this huge complex variability and work within that, rather than trying to strip it down to its individual components, where we start to lose sight of the big picture."

Another important thing to consider when it comes to using cannabis for pain is its relative safety when compared to other drugs that are usually the first line of defense for pain management. In 2015, Ware and a team of researchers published the COM-PASS study (Cannabis for the Management of Pain: Assessment of Safety Study), which was, to their knowledge, the first study on the long-term safety of medical cannabis.[15]

"I'd like to think I was sort of pushing for this [study] back then because there were increasing numbers of patients using cannabis legally at the time," Ware says, recalling that just one strain was available to patients through a single licensed producer operated by Health Canada. "It bothered me that it was being sent out to patients, but there was no attempt to follow up with the patients," he says.

Conducted between 2004 and 2008, the study comprised 431 subjects, with 215 using cannabis and 216 in the control group. Among the subjects using cannabis, most received an average daily dose of 2.5 grams of cannabis containing 12.5 percent THC. The study's authors note that in looking at "significant adverse events" that occurred during the study, the risk of having one such event was not significantly different between the two groups. The same was found for non-serious adverse events.

Another area of Ware's study that might surprise readers was his team's findings on the neuro-cognitive effects of cannabis use for pain: Both the cannabis users and the control group improved significantly on neurocognitive tests after six and twelve months of participating in the study. Pulmonary function tests also showed no significant changes after one year of cannabis use. Blood tests, though not conducted in all subjects of the study, showed that seventy-eight of the subjects had no changes in liver, renal, or endocrine function.

Of course, the efficacy measures of cannabis are arguably the most important aspect of the study. Subjects in the cannabis group noted a significant reduction in average pain intensity over the course of one year. (This reduction was not noted in the control group.) The cannabis users also indicated greater improvement in general physical function, a reduced sensory component of fear, and a significant improvement with regard to mood disturbances. Additionally, they reported feeling less anxious, depressed, angry, or fatigued than their control counterparts in the study.

"When you put it all together, what we found was that cannabis was remarkably well tolerated," Ware says.

Still, he stresses that it's important for patients who have been on other medications not to expect cannabis to be a panacea. It's one of the first things he tells patients when they come to him looking to cannabis as a solution to their chronic pain. "The first thing is to potentially dial down the expectations," he says. "With people who have chronic pain, there's often a very high hope that cannabis will be a treatment where everything else has failed. It's one approach like many others, and whether there's a benefit or not, we can find out together."

Using Cannabis for Pain Management

WARE SAYS THAT in most cases cannabis is considered a third line of attack for pain-related syndromes and symptoms, with opioids often being doctors' second choice and nonsteroidal anti-inflammatory drugs (NSAIDs) their first. It can be hard for patients to access cannabis before being directed to use other drugs, unless they convey to their physician that they'd like to take a more herbal approach, as it were.

"If you are a patient saying, 'Do I have to go through trials of opioids before I get to try cannabinoids?'—that's a pretty hot discussion right now in the medical community," he says. "Is it really necessary for somebody to have tried and failed opioid therapy before we try a drug like a cannabinoid? I think, no question, it has a far more favorable safety profile."

Ware takes his patients through an intake process that asks all the usual questions: the cause of the pain, what treatments have been tried and whether they've been effective, and what sort of side effects a patient has dealt with. Other questions more specific to cannabis treatment are whether a patient has a history of psychosis in the family, or if there is a historical or active substance use issue. Ware says an unstable heart or arrhythmias would also make a clinician "very cautious" about prescribing a cannabinoid drug.

"If all goes well and the patient understands that there is no guarantee that the benefits will be profound, and that there could be some side effects (like drowsiness, euphoria, or anxiety), a cautious trial of therapy would be indicated." Once a patient begins using cannabis to treat pain, Ware says he tries to work with them to determine what works most effectively, but says that there is no universal cannabinoid therapy for people who suffer from chronic pain.

Dr. Bryn Hyndman is the leading physician at Qi Integrated Health in Vancouver, B.C. With dual training as both an MD and a naturopathic doctor, Hyndman applies a functional medicine approach that integrates Western medicine and alternative therapies. She embraces cannabis as a relatively safe option for her patients, and recognizes that that separates her from other physicians, some of whom are apprehensive about recommending it.

"Most medical practitioners and physicians are not aware of or knowledgeable about the medicinal effects of cannabis, and that's because in medical school and residency, it's not in the curriculum," she tells me. Like many physicians I've spoken with who are of the mind that cannabis is in fact a medicine, Hyndman was first turned on to the idea by her patients. "They shared stories of incredible success using cannabis for chronic pain, acute pain, joint pain, sleep, anxiety, nerve pain, and in some cases mood disorders—it was really life-changing for them," she says. Because of her background in naturopathy and her understanding of medicinal plants, it made sense to her that cannabis would be used in this way by her patients. While she doesn't consider herself a pain specialist, she says about one-third of her patients use cannabis to treat pain.

When a patient comes to her in search of a remedy, Hyndman's process is similar to Ware's: she'll find out what other drugs they've tried, how effective those drugs have been, what sort of side effects the patient may have suffered from, and whether they prefer a pharmaceutical option. She says in some cases she'll be the one to suggest cannabis to her patients first, but there are certainly occasions where patients come in with a positive past experience with cannabis, and simply ask for approval to obtain their cannabis from a licensed producer.

In the process of narrowing down effective doses, cannabinoid ratios, and consumption methods for each patient, Hyndman regards cannabis as "just like any medication, supplement, or herb," in that there isn't a single regimented dose that will work for everyone. "The response is very individual," she says.

When it comes to managing pain, Hyndman says it's important to have both THC and CBD present in a medication so that they can work synergistically. "What I always recommend is to start at the lowest-dose THC possible, and preferably, to start in the evening and on a weekend when they don't have to work the next day, so they know how cannabis will make them feel," she says. For the most part, she says her patients are not interested in the euphoria that comes with THC, and so prefer to avoid it. "We have patients come in and say, 'I smoked a joint forty years ago but I don't want to get high now,'" she says. "I often tell them, 'It's about getting help, not getting high.'"

Hyndman says topicals can be a very effective way of treating acute pain, joint pain, or strained muscles, and are virtually free of side effects—though, depending on where you live in the world, these products might be unregulated. She warns her patients that edible cannabis products (such as an oil, tincture, capsule, or infused food) can take longer to kick in, but also have longer-lasting effects—sometimes more than eight hours.

While she says patients are moving away from smoking and even vaporizing, she recognizes that vaporizing provides a rapid onset of relief for acute pain that capsules or oils just don't provide.

A POWERFUL SUPPORT FOR CANCER TREATMENT

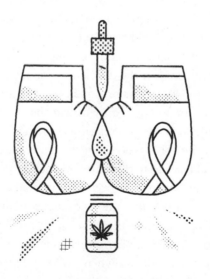

Case Study: Alan Park

BEING DIAGNOSED WITH cancer at age fifty-one was the last thing Canadian comedian Alan Park was expecting when he visited the doctor in 2013 to find out what was behind the nagging pain in his ribs. It turned out the unrelenting pain was symptomatic of stage four prostate cancer. His doctors advised him to begin a treatment that would suppress his body's ability to manufacture testosterone, the hormone that was fueling his cancer, but he was offered little else in the way of medicine.

At the time, the highly concentrated cannabis oils that are popular among cancer patients today weren't on the market. Park had heard about the value of cannabis for cancer patients, and so he did what many people do when they're told that they have just months to live: he decided to make his own. Using large amounts of dried cannabis, a solvent, and heat, Park carefully undertook the massive and potentially dangerous job and didn't look back.

"My feeling was, 'I need to get this done so that I can live,'" Park tells me by phone from Toronto. Upon his return to see a prostate surgeon specialist five weeks after his diagnosis, he was offered no further treatment, and was even told he was "too far gone" for chemotherapy, radiation, or surgery.

"When I went to see him, I'd already been taking cannabis for five weeks, and I'd experienced my own personal awareness of being in less pain," Park says. "I kept getting better and feeling better.... The specialist told me I didn't have any options, but I had already experienced an incredible markup in my quality of life."

That was around Christmas. By the following June, Park's physician had begun scratching his head. "I just don't understand," he said to Park. "You're doing so well!"

"I kept it from him for about five months, because I knew I was on to something, but to be honest, I wasn't sure if he would be okay with it," Park says. His hunch proved correct: upon telling his specialist about the wildcard that was at play, his physician advised against the continued use of cannabis oils that had not just improved Park's life, but also extended it.

Park chalked it up to a lack of knowledge on the doctor's part and proceeded to dig up doctor- and peer-reviewed studies and publications dating back to the 1970s, detailing the efficacy of cannabis as a treatment not just for the side effects associated with cancer but also for the cancer itself.

Today, Park is alive and his cancer is in remission. He goes for quarterly check-ups and tests, and he says his last several examinations have come back with "perfect" markers. He continues to use cannabis oil daily, but is now able to purchase it from a manufacturer and no longer makes his own.

Combining his ability as a comic with his passion for the healing properties of cannabis, Park hosts a weekly cannabis-focused podcast called *Green Crush*, which he uses to help disseminate information about the powerful characteristics of cannabis. "*Green* is the cannabis, and *crush* is what it does to cancer," he says.

For Park, the life-saving secret is one he simply can't keep to himself. "It's simple," he says. "I was refused all three doors, and I found another door. I just want to show people that there's one more door—that you can get to this place, and it's not dead."

Cancer: What It Is and How It Affects Us

....

I'M WILLING TO bet not a single person reading this book hasn't been affected by cancer in some way. Whether you've watched a friend struggle through chemotherapy and radiation, or you've had to say goodbye to a parent or grandparent sooner than expected, it's a disease (actually, a collection of related diseases) that mostly affects people over the age of fifty, but can occur at any age. The latest data from the American Cancer Society suggests 40 percent of men and 38 percent of women in the United States will develop cancer at some point in their lives,[1] with an expected 609,640 deaths to be caused by cancer in 2018.[2] In Canada, one in two people will develop cancer in their lifetime, and one in four will die from it, with Statistics Canada estimating that over 80,000 Canadians died of cancer in 2017.[3]

Though often referred to as a single disease, there are more than a hundred types of cancer. But from leukemia to melanoma, and breast cancer to prostate cancer, they all begin in the same way. Cancer starts at a cellular level, when cells in the tissues of our body begin to act abnormally, growing, working, and dividing—but not dying, like normal cells should. A buildup of these abnormal cells can form a tumor, though tumors are not a characteristic of every type of cancer. Tumors that are not cancerous are termed benign, and once they've been removed, it's unlikely that they'll come back. A malignant tumor, however, may return because cancerous cells can travel through other parts of the body— say, through the bloodstream—and spread to other areas. This is why early detection of cancer is so important.

The physical effects of cancer can vary from one person to the next, even if two people have the same type of cancer. Fatigue, pain, nausea, change in appetite, sleep problems, and a lack of interest in sex are all common side effects, but not everyone with cancer will experience them. Life-saving treatments like chemotherapy and radiation are physically demanding and can exacerbate these symptoms exponentially. The combined effect of cancer and cancer treatment on the body is certainly debilitating, but the effect of a cancer diagnosis on the mind is equally damaging. A cancer diagnosis significantly increases a person's risk of developing anxiety and depression and often leaves patients with a feeling of hopelessness and grief that seems insurmountable.

Common cancer treatments include chemotherapy, which uses a series of drugs to kill cancer cells, and radiation, which uses high-energy waves like X-rays, gamma rays, or charged particles to destroy or damage cancer cells. While these standard treatments are certainly effective, they also damage healthy cells in the body, and, as stated earlier, can add to and exacerbate the side effects of the cancer. Targeted therapy is another treatment that is used to block the action of certain enzymes, proteins, or molecules that are involved in the spread of cancer, while hormone therapy adds, blocks, or removes hormones to help stop cancer cells from continuing to reproduce, or to slow their reproduction. Treatment is certainly not limited to these four methods, though, with patients often supplementing them with complementary and alternative medicines to help improve their quality of life.

Historical Use of Cannabis for Cancer

OUR UNDERSTANDING OF how cancer works is relatively young. Some early theories, like German pathologist Johannes Müller's blastema theory, proposed that cancer did not come from normal cells. Others theorized that cancer was caused by chronic irritation or trauma, or that it was an infectious disease that was spread from person to person through parasites.[4] It wasn't until the middle of the twentieth century that scientists were able to understand how cancer manifests itself in the body; however, they still aren't quite sure what triggers cells in the body to act irregularly. This means our understanding of cannabinoid therapy in the context of cancer is also rather immature—but understanding how cancer operates wasn't necessary for historical cannabis users who found it to be an effective treatment for tumors and cancer-related symptoms.

Cannabis has been used historically over thousands of years to treat some of the *symptoms* associated with cancer and cancer treatment—records of it being used for nausea, lack of appetite, pain, sleep, inflammation, mood, and more can be found in ancient texts like the *Shennong Ben Cao Jing* and the sacred Hindu Vedas—but nailing down its historical use for cancer *as a disease* is a little more challenging. In his study "History of Cannabis and Its Preparations in Saga, Science, and Sobriquet," Dr. Ethan Russo refers to the Fayyum medical papyrus, a compilation of ancient Egyptian medical knowledge written sometime around the second half of the second century CE.

One entry speaks of "another (prescription) for curing the tumor," a method of pressing cannabis into a fine powder, mixing it with other herbs, including papyrus, lotus leaf, and sweet clover, and then applying it directly to a tumor and wrapping it with a bandage. A second entry describes a treatment of "paralyzing" tumors by mixing cannabis and other herbs into an extract before applying heat to the mixture and then to the affected area. Russo writes that the recommendation to apply heat is particularly interesting given that we know heat—or decarboxylation—converts THCA to THC. (See Chapter 5 for an explanation of decarboxylation.)

According to Russo, the next mention of cannabis as a treatment option for tumors did not arise until 1640. Herbalist John Parkinson wrote of using "fresh juice" of cannabis roots "mixed with a little

[oil] or butter" to help treat "hard tumors" in his book *Theatrum Botanicum: The Theatre of Plants*. Then, in 1758, French magistrate M. Marcandier wrote of the benefit of cannabis for tumors in his book, *Traité du chanvre* (available in English as *A Treatise on Hemp*): "The seed and the green leaves, crushed and applied in the form of cataplasm, to painful tumors, appear to be strongly resolutive and intoxicating," reads a translation of his method.[5]

In 1975, Albert E. Munson conducted the first study of cannabis as a potential cancer treatment in the *Journal of the National Cancer Institute*. Surprisingly, Munson found that when THC was administered to mice with malignant tumors in their lungs, the tumors stopped growing.[6] A few years later, in 1980, the National Cancer Institute began distributing a synthetic version of THC called Marinol to cancer patients in San Francisco. While some patients responded well to the synthetic medicine, studies being conducted in other parts of the United States that compared the use of the oral THC to smoked cannabis revealed that patients found smoked cannabis to be both safer and more effective.[7] Rather than considering the results of the studies that compared smoked cannabis to Marinol, the U.S. government opted to proceed with the synthetic version of the drug, leaving cannabis itself a Schedule I illegal narcotic and eventually approving Marinol as a Schedule II drug, meaning that it was considered to have "a high potential for abuse," in 1985. (It's since been moved to Schedule III, which means it's classified as having "moderate to low potential" for dependency.)[8] Marinol was prescribed for nausea and vomiting associated with chemotherapy. Despite the continued call from doctors and judges to remove cannabis from Schedule I and allow it as a medicinal treatment for cancer and chemotherapy symptoms, it took eleven years before the state of California enacted legislation that would allow cancer patients to use cannabis.

How Cannabis Can Help

DISCUSSING THE RELATIONSHIP between cannabis and cancer takes a bit of finesse. While cannabis has been considered a beneficial form of treatment for cancer and its symptoms for several decades, droves of so-called cannabis consultants and self-made Internet gurus—"Dr. Facebook," if you will—have spread some serious misinformation about cannabis and cancer. Worse, this information is not only untrue, it also has the potential to cause added harm to patients who are likely already suffering with the effects of a terminal illness.

As the founder of several companies that specialize in developing bio-pharmaceutical grade cannabinoid medicines for seriously ill patients and providing them with cannabis-specific services,

Mara Gordon knows a thing or two about how cannabis interacts with cancer cells. A researcher with a background in process engineering, she started her first company, Aunt Zelda's, in 2011 after losing several family members to cancer. At the time, she said she knew of the benefits of using cannabis to counteract the side effects of cancer, but when a patient with prostate cancer approached her and asked to use high doses of cannabis for its "cancer-killing" capabilities, she wasn't so sure.

"I had read about the Rick Simpson oil and the protocol of a gram a day to, quote-unquote, 'cure' any type of cancer, and it was so preposterous that I was skeptical about how to proceed," she says. After reading the preclinical trials, though, Gordon says her eyes were opened to the plant's healing possibilities—but she maintains that using the word "cure" to describe the effects of cannabis on cancer is not only misleading, it's flat-out wrong. "Our experience has been that as soon as patients stop using cannabis, the tumors return. How can you say something is a cure if you have to continue treatment?"

People may get the impression from survivor stories or even news articles that because cannabinoids actually do "kill" cancer cells (I'll get to how in a minute), that somehow makes cannabis a cure for the disease—but as Gordon said, any treatment that has to continue indefinitely is certainly not a cure in the traditional sense of the word. But not using that particular word to describe the process of what cannabis does to the body doesn't make it any less remarkable: Gordon explains that when activated, the endocannabinoid receptors located throughout the body (both CB1 and CB2) destroy cells by inducing something called *apoptosis*, or "cell suicide."

"This occurs within the body while protecting the healthy cells from the damaging effects of chemotherapy and radiation," she says.

This is shown in a 2017 study published in the *Journal of Exploratory Research in Pharmacology*, which notes that while cannabis has been used in the palliative treatment of cancer for a long time, advancements in research on the endocannabinoid system have shown that cannabinoids can be effective anti tumor agents because of "their ability to induce apoptosis... and promote cell growth inhibition." It notes that since 1975, several studies have found that cannabinoids induce apoptosis in both *in vitro* models (in a petri dish) and *in vivo* (in living organisms), and lists several publications that report successfully treating aggressive tumors in this way. The authors also write that "the concentration of cannabinoid receptors on tumor cells has been found to be much higher than on the corresponding normal tissue," and state that while both CB1 and CB2 receptors play a role in halting cancer in its tracks, the receptor that is thought to be primarily responsible for triggering apoptosis—cell suicide—is CB2.[9]

One thing that makes cannabinoid treatment for cancer so appealing to physicians and oncologists is that it is able to protect healthy cells in the body while slowing tumor growth and killing cancer cells. And that's not all. Gordon says preliminary data shows that cannabis can have a synergistic effect on traditional cancer treatments like chemotherapy and radiation, making them work more effectively. One study Gordon references found that when researchers combined THC with temozolomide, a chemotherapy drug used to treat brain tumors, the two agents enhanced each other's ability to induce cell death in a glioma, or brain tumor.[10] This has been shown to be extremely useful for tumors that become resistant to chemotherapy.[11] But Gordon warns that genetic differences from patient to patient mean that combining chemotherapy with cannabis is by no means guaranteed to work. "That isn't always the case," she says, "because you could have ten people with the same diagnosis, and they each have their own genetic anomaly that's associated with their particular type of cancer, and it may or may not work for them."

Using Cannabis for Cancer

LET'S GET HYPOTHETICAL for a second: you've just been diagnosed with cancer. Trust what I'm about to say, and know that it's been echoed by every cancer expert I've ever spoken with on this topic: do not, I repeat, do not immediately send yourself down an Internet rabbit hole on a search for a cannabis "cure" for your diagnosis. Odds are, you'll come across some conflicting advice—from articles advising you to start taking massive amounts of high-THC oil "and nothing else" for several months, to others claiming cannabis has absolutely no medical benefit for cancer patients. The truth lies somewhere in the middle. As wonderful as cannabis is in this context, we can't overlook the role that chemotherapy and radiation play in cancer treatment.

"If you have a type of cancer and doctors say 70 percent of the patients that have done standard chemo and radiation have gone into remission after five years, you'd be *out of your mind* to not do chemo and radiation," says Gordon when I ask about the inherent risks associated with listening to the advice of those she refers to as Dr. Facebook.

"If a doctor says, 'Well, we don't have anything for this, but we can try chemo and it's about 20 percent'—even then, you'd be crazy not to try, because if you do it along with cannabinoids it may increase your chances. It's not that if you use a natural way of treatment that you can't do the other, and that's the message that so much of the Internet puts out there. It's my personal pet peeve... you can't swing a cat without hitting a [so-called] cannabis guru." Not only that, Gordon says there's an added risk in attempting to complete some of the protocols: they often recommend very high amounts of THC, which could lead unknowing patients to believe that if they can't handle the high dose, cannabis isn't an option for them at all.

Your ability to access cannabis and use it in conjunction with a more conventional treatment will certainly depend on your location. While medical cannabis is becoming legal in different countries around the world at an increasing rate, the plant is still considered medically ineffective in other parts of the world.

Let's get hypothetical again, and assume you're living in a part of the world where medical cannabis is accessible. Even in those places, Gordon says one of the biggest obstacles to accessing cannabis for cancer-related reasons is the idea that cannabis treatment requires customization for each patient. She says while this notion often leads doctors away from suggesting cannabis because they feel they lack the time or expertise to tailor the treatment to their patient, it's no different from the customization required for pharmaceuticals. "With pharmaceuticals, the doctor doesn't really have to be an active participant in decision making—it's like, 'First you try this, then you try that.' Cannabis doesn't have that road map out there for physicians right now, so the doctor has to be involved," says Gordon. Without knowledge of the complexities of the plant's compounds and how they work synergistically in the body, navigating cannabis treatment for cancer is likely a scary thought for a physician.

It's why Gordon calls cannabis "participatory medicine": the doctor has to be an active participant in patient care—the other end of the spectrum of what has become the standard of care in North America, where most doctor visits last just twenty minutes at most.[12]

At the California practice Gordon founded, Calla Spring Wellness, she says the physicians there have developed somewhat of a road map for cancer patients. Depending on the type of cancer the patient has been diagnosed with, Gordon says they'll work to target the cannabinoid receptors that are more commonly found in the area affected by the cancer. (Check out Appendix 1 to learn where CB1 and CB2 receptors are located throughout the body.) "The first thing we do is we look at the part of the body and the type of cancer.... If it's a central nervous system–type cancer, whether it's in the spine or it's a brain tumor, then it's CB1, and we'll try and tackle it with a higher level of THC and lower levels of CBD. But when we're dealing with patients and CB2 is the dominant receptor, we'll often go with a 1:1 or 1:2 ratio of THC to CBD."

Gordon says her team has also found certain profiles of plants that seem to not only work more effectively, but also be tolerated better by patients. She says these plants have terpene profiles that include linalool, limonene, myrcene, and, in particular, beta-caryophyllene—one of the very few noncannabinoid compounds that actually activates the CB2 receptor, she says. On the other hand, cultivars high in alpha- or beta-pinene have caused some patients discomfort, making it hard for them to comply with treatment because they don't like the feeling of the high. "The purples are interesting. If we think about the profiles of the plants that contain those terpenes I mentioned, often those are found in Granddaddy Purple, Grape Ape, Purple Urkle, or similar plants," she says.

Another finding Gordon and her team have made in their decades of treating cancer patients? She says there's likely no correlation between the weight of the patient and their required dose of cannabis. "You can't say milligrams per kilogram like you can with so many pharmaceuticals," she says. "We also find that most of the time women require a lower dose than men. There's a lot of customization that takes place; however, we're picking away at some of those obstacles so there is less customization that has to occur."

Using cannabis to treat the side effects of cancer and not the cancer itself requires a slightly less complicated road map and largely depends on your intention: Are you trying to quell nausea? Pain? Depression? Some patients laud Harlequin, a strain with about a 2:1 ratio of CBD to THC, for its ability to relieve pain, while others prefer heavier strains high in THC like Purple Kush or Trainwreck, which might be better suited to evening use. Other more uplifting varieties like Super Lemon Haze or Jillybean, perhaps better used during the day, can help with nausea and vomiting.

Just as the type of cannabis you're using will likely depend on the outcome you're looking for, so will your method of consumption. Faster relief from quick-onset nausea might be better served by vaporizing or smoking, while an unrelenting pain might be better tackled with a high-potency tincture or capsule. If you plan to use cannabis to try to treat your cancer, products like highly concentrated "tears" (a full extract oil often made with ethanol or grain alcohol) will provide you with a much higher cannabinoid content per dose, but these can induce a rather intense experience if you're not used to the euphoric effects that can come with consuming products that are high in cannabinoids. Be sure to talk to your doctor if you're considering this.

EASING THE
AGING PROCESS

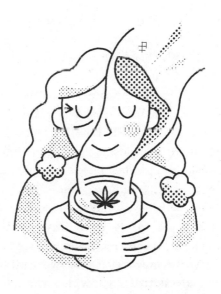

Case Study: Selena Wong

WHEN SELENA WONG began taking care of her elderly grandparents in her early twenties, she learned quickly that in times of extreme stress or anxiety, cannabis provided her with patience and understanding. "It's my sanity as a caregiver," she tells me by phone from her home in Vernon, B.C., where she operates Flower of Life Integrative Health. "I never had kids, so stepping in to take care of two majorly dependent people was a whole other challenge."

Wong says that every day she'd go for her sanity toke, a quick puff to relax—and she soon found herself wondering if cannabis could provide her oma and opa with as much relief as she was getting from the herb. She started small with a medicated jam to help her grandmother through something called sundowning, a symptom of dementia that can cause increased confusion and restlessness. Wong says the "special" jam allowed her grandmother to have more restful sleeps and seemed to restore some of her lucidity. "Every morning, her cognition was better," she says. "Sometimes she was verbal, and other times not, but after we used the special jam, she would wake up clearer, more rested and confident, and she was able to communicate more effectively. It was amazing to watch."

She describes that the cannabis revealed a truer, more authentic version of her oma, as her learned behaviors began to fall away and familiar, more youthful parts of her personality shone through. "I found this joyous, relaxed, calm, confident woman, even when she was going through a struggle," she says.

While her oma struggled with Alzheimer's and dementia, her opa maintained clarity of mind but struggled with pain that made sleeping very difficult. "When we started with my oma, my opa noticed that she was having these great sleeps. He was having a hard time with his prostate, had limited mobility, and needed help all the time." It wasn't long before Wong was giving her grandfather special jam before bed too, and soon he was sleeping through the night. Despite his deeply ingrained belief that cannabis was "evil," Wong says she was able to communicate its benefits to him in a way that opened his mind to the possibility of using it.

"When we started talking about marijuana putting you to sleep, he started to rethink that relationship," she says.

On his deathbed, Selena says, her grandfather was in too much pain to eat or drink—but he'd still ask for the infused jam. When Selena's grandmother passed away several years later, cannabis was at play once again, easing the transition from life to death for her grandmother and also helping family members through the grieving process. "Having cannabis as an ally at the end of life, in my opinion, is one of the most valuable allies you can have," Wong says. "Cannabis has the ability to bring a sense of peace, so when people are going through that death process—the death of the ego, the personality, the anxiety—cannabis can help through that struggle."

Aging: Not Just the Body Getting Older

AS MUCH AS we humans know aging is inevitable, we'll do just about anything to try to stop it in its tracks—from normal things like applying sunscreen and eating healthy foods to more drastic endeavors like getting placenta facials or having blood injections, à la Kim Kardashian. Of course, aging goes far beyond the physical—and frankly, I'm more interested in what I can do to protect myself from Alzheimer's disease, stroke, or, say, knee replacements than a few laugh lines or crow's-feet. From arthritis to dementia to Parkinson's disease, the list of illnesses associated with aging is long, and the symptoms of such diseases can have detrimental effects on a person's quality of life, especially if they're being affected by more than one illness at a time, which is often the case.

It's no secret that the elderly are the fastest-growing demographic of cannabis users in the United States—as reported by the *New Yorker*, the *Globe and Mail*, CBS, and just about every other major publication and television network in North America. In 2017, the U.S. Census Bureau confirmed that the population of seniors in the United States was growing. Across Canada, the population of seniors also continues to grow. Statistics Canada estimates that the nation's 65+ demographic will exceed 18 percent of the population by 2021—up more than 4 percent from ten years earlier. This trend in population growth is already forcing us to think outside of the pharmaceutical box when it comes to how we might treat our grandparents, parents, and elders.

Depending on our genetics and the kind of lives we've led, we all age at different rates: everyone knows at least one seventy-year-old who enjoys going for long walks, heading out with friends to social events, and engaging in activities that some fifty-year-olds we know would never dare try unless a La-Z-Boy and a football game were involved. While everyone's muscles will age, shrink, and lose mass, a person who has lived a more active life will lose muscle more slowly than someone who has regularly spent five out of seven nights in front of the tube. As we age, our bones lose mineral content, and the lubrication in our joints and tendons is reduced, making it harder to move as swiftly as we might have in our twenties or thirties. Our hearts, too, become weaker. Our metabolisms slow as well, which can sometimes lead to weight gain. (This stops when the rate of weight gain is outpaced by the loss of lean muscle, usually around age fifty-five for men and sixty-five for women.) This is not a book about exercise, but it is a book about health—and since we're going to talk about making aging easier, I'll be so bold as to say that physical activity is most certainly one of the *best* things you can do to make getting older a less miserable process. Other important but obvious ones include eating a healthy diet rich in vegetables, healthy fats, and protein; managing stress; and getting quality sleep.

Other aspects of aging affect our brain function and cognition—memory loss by way of Alzheimer's disease and dementia is very common, with an estimated fifty million people around the world living with dementia in 2017, according to Alzheimer's Disease International.[1] The organization estimates that the number will double every twenty years.

Historical Use of Cannabis for Aging
....

ALTHOUGH THEY MAY not have been as concerned with the shift in demographics currently facing our society, it's highly likely that our ancestral cannabis users benefited from the anti-aging effects of cannabis without even knowing it. Lise Manniche wrote in her 1985 book, *An Ancient Egyptian Herbal*, that cannabis was used to treat glaucoma, an age-related disease affecting the eyes. Jonathon Green writes in *Cannabis*, his 2002 book, that as early as 600 BCE, cannabis was used in India to "quicken the mind" and "prolong life."[2] It's likely that among the more than one hundred ailments cannabis was recommended for as a treatment in the *Shennong Ben Cao Jing*, at least some were age-related. When Nicholas Culpeper wrote about cannabis in *The English Physician*, he lauded it for its ability to treat "knots in the joints" and "the pains of the sinews and hips"[3]—suggesting relief from arthritis. When cannabis became popularized in the mid-1800s and was added to the *U.S. Pharmacopeia*, it was listed as a treatment for several conditions, including gout and incontinence. The Indian Hemp Drugs Commission of 1894 made similar findings.

How Cannabis Can Help

. . . .

SOME MIGHT SCRATCH their heads as to why more and more seniors are deciding to supplement their medication with cannabis (or in many cases substitute it completely), but the rest of us know that given the numerous uses for cannabis just described in this little book—trust me, there are many more—it's no wonder an increasing number of our elders are opting to use it.

Think about the afflictions the elderly in our lives often deal with. Pain and cancer are two areas that make up a considerable number of conditions affecting seniors, and are part of the reason why cannabis is gaining so much popularity among this group—cannabis can provide relief from multiple ailments at once! In addition to experiencing chronic pain or cancer, a person approaching the end of their life might feel anxiety, fear, or depression, and cannabis can work wonders when it comes to putting those feelings into perspective. In fact, caregivers often report that end-of-life cannabis use helps elderly patients reconcile with the fact that they're about to die. And if we think back to the importance of sleep and the way a good night's rest can in many instances be made better with a little cannabis, we can see how several topics already covered can lend themselves to cannabis use among seniors.

There are other areas to consider, including the neurological changes that come with aging and the effects of Alzheimer's disease or dementia (which, to be clear, is not a single disease but a class of symptoms marked by memory loss and a decline in thinking skills). A few studies have shown that cannabis may help to manage behavioral symptoms associated with these conditions. A 2017 literature review published in the journal *Current Neurology and Neuroscience Reports* found that in previous literature, while synthetic THC proved to be just as effective as other medications used for dementia, several case studies found that it was a superior medicine. The authors of the study said that given the other benefits associated with cannabis use, it was a better treatment for behavioral issues associated with dementia than conventional medications like antipsychotics, which have been shown to increase the risk of mortality due to cardiovascular events as well as aspiration (accidentally breathing in foreign matter).[4]

Other research seems to point in the direction that cannabis could not just assist with the symptoms of dementia, but also help prevent it from developing in the first place. (I know there are at least a few of you reading who might associate cannabis use with increased forgetfulness, and while I can certainly relate—I've definitely smoked a little too much sticky-icky and temporarily misplaced my keys before—the research doesn't lie.) A preclinical study published in the *Journal of Alzheimer's Disease* in 2014 investigated whether THC had therapeutic potential for preventing a hallmark characteristic of Alzheimer's disease: the development of beta-amyloid proteins, which can build up and create plaques in the brain.[5] The researchers found that THC was able to slow the production of beta-amyloid proteins, which form the plaques that block signaling in the brain. An earlier study, published in the journal *Molecular Pharmaceutics* in 2006, had come to a similar conclusion: "THC and its analogues may provide an improved therapeutic for Alzheimer's disease... simultaneously treating both the symptoms and the progression of Alzheimer's disease."[6] As impressive as this may sound, it's just the tip of the proverbial neurodegenerative iceberg when it comes to cannabis. In 2016, scientists at the Salk Institute in California were able to demonstrate in preliminary findings that cannabinoids—in addition to serving as both a treatment and prevention—could also actively reduce the amount of beta-amyloid already present in the brain, while putting a stop to the inflammatory response it created.[7]

You might also recall the publicity around a study published by researchers from the University of Bonn in 2017, which suggested that cannabis could reverse the aging process in the brain. Though it was conducted on mice, often the first stage in such cutting-edge research, the results are promising. Lead researcher Dr. Andreas Zimmer and his team were able to show that with prolonged low-dose treatment of THC, older mice "regressed" to the state of younger mice. After THC was regularly administered to mice aged two, twelve, and eighteen months, learning capacity and memory performance of the mice were tested. While the mice that were given a placebo continued to show signs of aging at a regular rate, regardless of their age, the twelve- and eighteen-month-old mice that were given THC eventually had the cognitive performance of two-month-old mice.[8] Zimmer reported that the treatment "completely reversed the loss of performance in the old animals."

Using Cannabis to Ease Aging

ONE RESEARCHER WITH a deep understanding of not just how seniors land on the notion of cannabis use but also how their doctors warm up to the idea of prescribing it is Dr. Brian Kaskie, an associate professor in the Department of Health Management and Policy at the University of Iowa. Kaskie has a particular interest in public policy as it affects the elderly, and has worked in this area for twenty-five years.

Let's rewind to the point I mentioned earlier in this chapter that seniors are the fastest-growing demographic of cannabis users in North America. In 2017, Kaskie and a team of researchers published a study that questioned if such an increase in cannabis use should be considered "a public health crisis or viable policy alternative."[9] They took a close look at the factors that affect a senior's decision to use cannabis, what they were primarily using it for, and whether such use could lead to unexpected harms.

Kaskie determined that rather than being the potential cause of a health crisis, cannabis could very well be an alternative that supports the health and well-being of seniors in a way that is more effective and less harmful than standard medications. But most physicians in the United States aren't trained to work with cannabinoids and aren't exactly ready to consider recommending a federally illegal drug to their patients. A few, he says, will initiate the conversation, but in most cases, it's up to the patient to request cannabis as an alternative to conventional medicine. This barrier is something Kaskie says policy makers should consider as they search for ways to tackle the opioid crisis, a health epidemic that has resulted in an astounding number of deaths affecting all ages, races, and classes, and that shows no signs of abating.

"The evidence from our focus groups and surveys say this is pretty big," he says, noting that older women are the largest population group in the

United States seeking opioid prescriptions. "When they're prescribed appropriately and managed, they certainly do have their place in care. However, even among the older adults, the enthusiasm to prescribe opioids is far in excess of the actual need for it."

Kaskie says overprescription of medication to nursing home residents—a common problem in the 1970s and '80s, he says—is seeing a resurgence. It's one of the reasons he thinks there's a need to consider alternatives to opioids and other prescription drugs in the specific context of seniors. Older patients told Kaskie and his team that not only did they find that cannabis relieved their pain, it also served as an effective replacement for prescription drugs that may have been diminishing their quality of life. Of course, he notes that the lack of federal approval of cannabis as a medicinal substance means the adoption of such an idea by the medical community will take time.

While physicians who work with seniors and cannabis do exist, there isn't exactly a guide to prescribing cannabis for geriatric patients, though one might assume that smoking isn't the best option for an elderly person. "I have to admit, I thought the only way you could have it was to smoke it," Kaskie says, "but that's not true. There are creams and gummies and all these different ways to take it. We found a lot of seniors also didn't know, and yet, when they found out, they said, 'Oh, well, I'll take it that way.'" He adds that the stereotype of smoking a joint or smoking a pipe has "done a lot" to create the negative association that many seniors have with cannabis.

Speaking specifically about palliative care and end-of-life treatment, Kaskie says that because cannabis can effectively relieve a variety of symptoms, it can provide patients with an opportunity to die at home if they prefer. "If you're at the end of life, and you're experiencing nausea, or pain, and this substance works for you, why not? It's a great alternative to being in the hospital and having all sorts of treatments that you don't need," he says, adding that four medical cannabis state programs have made cannabis available for end-of-life care. "These state programs, it's not the teenagers who are showing up for these programs, it's the older adults."

While some physicians say prescribing cannabis to an older adult puts them at greater risk of certain negative outcomes, like an increased chance of heart attack for those with pre-existing heart conditions, or an increased likelihood of falling, Kaskie says the risks are relatively low. "When we ask older adults in our self-reported surveys, 'What are the outcomes here?' we get very, very few older adults saying, 'Things are getting worse,' or 'I've had more accidents,' or 'I've gone to the emergency room more times,'" Kaskie says. "As a researcher who is sort of agnostic about all of this, this is interesting to me because it's a story that counters everything we're hearing in the general research literature." The incongruence begins to make sense when we consider that the number of seniors represented in existing cannabis research is far lower than the number of eighteen- to thirty-five-year-olds, he says.

Based on Kaskie's knowledge of how cannabis is being used among seniors in the United States, it's safe to say that while smoking could certainly be an option for those interested in doing so, by and large, seniors prefer alternative methods of consumption like tinctures, edibles, capsules, or topicals. As I've said many times before, a patient's intended outcome will often determine how they decide to consume. Seniors suffering from arthritis or pain confined to a certain area might prefer to start with an infused topical. (I have had great success introducing seniors to cannabis in this way, as it is the least intrusive method of consumption and often quite enjoyable.) A vaporizer pen can provide quick relief in instances of nausea or quick-onset pain, while edible forms of cannabis can provide longer-lasting relief. It's important to remember, though, that Grandma's metabolism definitely doesn't work as quickly as your own—edibles might take twice as long to kick in for a senior, and their effects might then last double the length of time they do for you.

Selena Wong, who was featured in this chapter's case study, has worked with numerous elderly patients at her integrative health clinic, and she says she tries to ensure that each and every one of them is introduced to cannabis in a warm and welcoming way. "I'm really mindful that the people I work with have a positive experience," she says. "I always start with topical lotions or CBD products, as they're nonintoxicating. Oftentimes, with the conditioning that seniors have experienced, it helps them reframe that relationship with the plant, without having a negative experience." Wong touts a whole-plant approach—even when using CBD products—over products made from single-cannabinoid distillations or isolated compounds. For seniors who have complex issues with swallowing, Wong suggests sublingual drops or sprays that can be easily administered.

Above all, though, Wong says the importance of having a senior's consent must be paramount: "If the senior is able to consent and understand, that's incredibly important. I would hate for a senior—say, in a home—to be given cannabis and have an experience that's not positive. Seniors are people, and just like you or I would want to know, so do they."

Based on her experiences with other seniors and, of course, with her own grandparents, Wong says cannabis can ease people into coming to terms with their own death in a way that other medicines just can't. "Having cannabis as an ally at the end of life is so valuable, because she has the ability to bring about a sense of peace," she says, referring to the feminized, flowering plant. "When people are going through the process, that fear, that unknown anxiety, it's a lot less when we're working with cannabis. It's like she invites you to the other realm of the universe."

THE EXIT DRUG

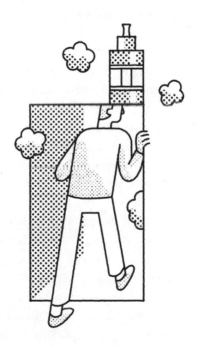

Case Study: Siobhan McCarthy
....

WHEN SIOBHAN MCCARTHY, a lifelong athlete and former national figure skating champion, was the victim of a major car accident that caused severe damage to her leg, it turned her life upside down. Following an intense surgery in which three of the ligaments in her knee were replaced, she was placed on an intravenous morphine drip, and she remembers being served a host of drug cocktails during her three-week stay in the hospital.

Not doing well on the medication, and unaware that she was becoming physically addicted to the drugs she was being prescribed, McCarthy said her doctors hadn't prepared her for what she was about to experience. At the time of the accident, she was twenty-two, an elite athlete studying political science and spending her vacations teaching skiing and sailing to put herself through school. After being released from the hospital, unable to walk, McCarthy fell into a major depression—so her doc- · tor added antidepressants to her growing list of medications. The cocktail of pharmaceuticals made for nightmarish side effects, including weight gain, extreme nausea, a feeling of emotional numbness and withdrawal, and, sometimes, lack of control over her bodily functions.

"Going from that, to all of a sudden being in a wheelchair and addicted to different medications—I was put on it all—it felt like I was being drugged to be complacent," she says. "My whole twenties were lost to getting better." When her surgeon suggested that McCarthy give cannabis a try, she made a conscious decision to start weaning herself off the host of addictive medications she'd been taking for more than five years. "I took myself off of everything, and I used cannabis to help me through that," she says.

While the antidepressants and opiates she had been taking numbed her to emotion, killed her appetite, and subdued her ability to speak up when doctors added yet another medication to her regimen, cannabis not only mitigated the pain in her leg, it also brought a sense of perspective to a mind that had been clouded by years of prescription medication. And while she describes the withdrawals as "hell on earth," cannabis helped to at least make them bearable.

"It helped me come to terms with the life that I thought I was going to have versus the life that I was having. It helped me to adjust ... and to listen to that tiny voice within, to reconnect with my sense of self, my body, and my healing process," she says.

Today, McCarthy is able to manage her pain with cannabis (as she has been doing for the last fifteen years), and she says it's responsible for more than just providing her with relief from pain and a way out of her addiction. It also helped her access her creativity: since the accident, she's embarked on a career in both the arts and the cannabis industry, becoming an accomplished playwright, filmmaker, and public relations professional. "Sometimes I wonder how I got through it all. All I can say is, thank God I found cannabis."

What Is Addiction?
....

THE AVERAGE PERSON might be able to consume a few alcoholic drinks without getting belligerent, or bet on a game of blackjack and know when to collect their chips and cash out, but when that pleasurable behavior becomes compulsive and begins to negatively interfere with life, it crosses the line into addiction. For the purposes of this book, we'll focus on the type of addiction that involves substance use.

An addicted brain essentially becomes rewired

to continue taking a substance despite the negative consequences that might be associated with doing so. Repeated drug use can affect the structure and function of the brain by altering the limbic system, which includes the brain's reward system, regulating feelings of pleasure. This system, an essential part of our survival, rewards behaviors that are good for us—like eating when we're hungry—so that we repeat those behaviors. But an addictive substance hijacks the limbic system by either mimicking or creating an overproduction of dopamine, a neurochemical that sends signals to the brain's reward system. This dopamine spike is what separates doing drugs from eating a tasty meal or having sex: while the latter activities release normal levels of the neurochemical, addictive substances flood the reward system with too much dopamine. Over time, the brain loses its ability to produce normal levels and only the addictive substance can activate the reward system.

In the current *Diagnostic and Statistical Manual of Mental Disorders* (DSM-5), a handbook used by healthcare professionals to diagnose conditions related to mental health, the American Psychiatric Association lays out eleven criteria for substance use disorders, including cravings and urges to use, taking more than the recommended dose for long periods of time, trying to cut back but being unable to do so, and continuing to use even in the face of the loss of personal relationships and interest in occupational or recreational activities.[1]

Between 1999 and 2016, more than 630,000 Americans died as a result of a drug overdose.[2] Researchers and physicians around the world are struggling to come up with more reliable and affordable ways to combat drug addiction in the face of overdose rates that don't seem to be slowing down. Drug replacement therapies, live-in treatment centers, and other common methods can be costly solutions for individuals if not covered by insurance or government funding, and especially for vulnerable populations who are often more susceptible to addiction. Even if people who are addicted to drugs are able to abstain, the likelihood of relapse is 40 to 60 percent, according to the National Institute on Drug Abuse (NIDA).

Opioid addiction in particular has affected North America more dramatically in the last five years than in any period since records began, with numbers continuing to rise each year. In the United States, the Centers for Disease Control and Prevention declared in June 2017 that overdoses had become the leading cause of death among Americans under the age of fifty[3]—increasing by 19 percent between 2015 and 2016, with at least 59,000 deaths in 2016—surpassing the highest annual death rates ever caused by car accidents, gun violence, or AIDS. In Western Canada, the cheap but potent opioid fentanyl has tainted, if not replaced, most of the street heroin supply, causing a greatly increased death rate among street drug users over the last five years. Not every province tracks overdose deaths, so it's hard to say how severe the problem has become on a national scale, but in B.C., the number of deaths rose 88 percent between 2016 and 2017.[4]

History of the "Exit Drug" Theory

IN THE PARTS of the continent where cannabis use has been either legalized or decriminalized, its consumption is increasingly seen as normal, but some continue to grip tightly onto ideas spread following the "Reefer Madness" era, which began in the 1930s. One notion in particular seems especially tough to overturn. The gateway drug theory is the idea that using one drug, particularly cannabis, can lead to an increased probability of using other, more harmful drugs. Although researcher Denise Kandel coined the term over forty years ago in a paper that discussed the dangers of nicotine, cannabis became the iconic gateway drug in the late 1970s when White House drug czar Robert DuPont vilified it as part of what is still known as the War on Drugs.

These days, scientists are learning that the evidence points in a very different direction. Not only has the gateway drug theory been repeatedly debunked, it could even be argued that it's been replaced with the notion of the "exit drug," which suggests that cannabis can be used to facilitate an end to a dependency on, and even addiction to, other, more dangerous drugs.

But before we explore the earliest expressions of this idea, let's consider from a common sense perspective why cannabis is, without a doubt, a safer alternative to more addictive substances. For one, cannabis has a higher margin of safety than legal substances like tobacco and alcohol, meaning the amount required to feel its effects is much smaller than the amount that would be toxic. Cannabis is also considered to be less physically addictive than alcohol or opioids, but it is important to note that some users do develop problematic use that can lead to dependence and symptoms like irritability, cravings, or difficulty sleeping. The risk of developing problematic use increases the younger a user begins consuming cannabis,[5] though plenty of people who consume cannabis in their youth don't go on to experience problematic use.[6] And while people who use cannabis should certainly be of a certain age and use it safely, no one has ever died from consuming cannabis.[7]

One of the first investigations into the idea that cannabis could be used as a substitute for other substances began around the same time that DuPont and other Republicans blamed cannabis for the nation's drug problem. In 1970, Dr. Tod Mikuriya published research in the *Psychedelic Review* that looked at the role of cannabis use in the recovery of patients with alcoholism.

"It would appear that for selected alcoholics the substitution of smoked cannabis for alcohol may be of marked rehabilitative value," he wrote. He also noted that cannabis didn't produce symptoms of irritability during withdrawal, or negative effects on the gastrointestinal tract.[8] In a review of research published in 1973, Mikuriya cites multiple nineteenth- and twentieth-century physicians who used cannabis to successfully treat opiate and chloral hydrate addictions, even writing that some preferred it because unlike opiates, cannabis use didn't lead to physical dependence.[9] All in all, he references fifty-six studies authored between 1857 and 1972 that indicate that cannabis has therapeutic potential as an anti-withdrawal agent for opiate and alcohol addiction. Unfortunately, the political climate of the time and the negative public perception of cannabis meant that much of Mikuriya's research went unnoticed. Today, the addiction treatment industry largely rejects the idea that cannabis has a place in the treatment of drug addiction, but health scientists following in Mikuriya's footsteps are eager to prove them wrong.

How Cannabis Can Help
....

DR. MIKURIYA MAY have been one of the first U.S. doctors to take an unbiased look at cannabis in the context of substitution for more addictive substances, but since the year 2000, internationally recognized cannabis expert and public health researcher Dr. Amanda Reiman has been considering the implications of his work.

Reiman has confirmed with her own research, over and over again, that whether physicians agree with the practice or not, adults are substituting cannabis for alcohol and other drugs— including prescription opioids. In one survey of medical cannabis dispensary users Reiman conducted in Berkeley, California, she found that of the 350 respondents, 40 percent used cannabis as a substitute for alcohol, while 26 percent used it in place of illicit drugs, and 66 percent chose cannabis over prescription drugs. A number of study participants responded positively to more than one category of substitution. Among their reasons for substituting, users said they preferred cannabis because they experienced fewer adverse side effects, better symptom management, and reduced withdrawal potential when compared with other drugs.[10]

Like any good researcher, Reiman knew the results had to be replicated, and in 2013, she worked with Canadian researchers on a study that looked at a slightly larger sample size. Of the 404 respondents, who used dispensaries in B.C., Canada, over 75 percent said they used cannabis in place of at least one other substance.[11] This was a factor in Reiman and her co-authors' concluding that scientists should consider conducting randomized clinical trials on cannabis substitutions for problematic substance use.

Reiman's latest research gets a little more specific by focusing on cannabis as a replacement for opioids. With 2,897 participants, the study boasts one of the largest-ever samples used for research on substitution, and it produced some astonishing statistics. A total of 97 percent of the sample "strongly agreed" or "agreed" that consuming cannabis allowed them to reduce their opioid consumption. Additionally, 92 percent said that the side effects of cannabis consumption were more tolerable than those of opioids, while 81 percent said that they found cannabis to be a more effective treatment than opioids. Taking the data a step further, 93 percent said that if cannabis were more readily available, they'd be more likely to use it for their condition.[12] As more and more jurisdictions legalize both medical and recreational cannabis use, Reiman's research lends support to the idea that increased access to cannabis could result in a reduction in overdose deaths. I'm sure no one would dispute that this research comes at a critical time.

Now before you brush off the notion that cannabis access can actually reduce the number of overdose deaths, consider the findings of a 2017 study that examined hospitalizations in the United States over a seventeen-year period. Researchers found that in states where medical marijuana was legal, fewer people were hospitalized for opioid use than in states where it was not. Hospitalizations caused by opioid dependence or abuse fell by 23 percent in states after they implemented medical marijuana policies, while hospitalizations caused by overdoses dropped by 13 percent.[13] Another recent study that looked specifically at the state of Colorado found that opioid-related deaths fell by nearly 7 percent in the two years following the state's decision to legalize recreational cannabis.[14]

Thanks to the work of scientists like Reiman, we've known for some time that cannabis is being used as a substitute for prescription drugs and alcohol, and patients actually prefer to use it rather than other drugs like opioids. Other researchers have taken cues from Reiman and have dug further into the idea that cannabis use might have implications in this area by looking closely at the role that the body's endocannabinoid system plays in the context of addiction, asking critical questions that examine the interactions at a neurochemical level.

A 2017 review article in the journal *Neuropharmacology* confirms the suspicion you might have by now that endocannabinoid signaling is involved in the system of reward, or the part of the brain known as the limbic system.[15] The authors of the paper reviewed the findings of randomized controlled trials that evaluated the efficacy of cannabinoid-based medications in treating addiction. Most medications specifically intended for treating addiction target the ECS by working on the body's CB1 receptors, which are found in the same regions of the brain where addictive behaviors are developed and maintained. (See Appendix 1.)

Because different substances affect the brain in different ways, scientists have had to consider each substance's interaction with the ECS separately. When it comes to alcohol, the study found that CBD could reduce consumption in mice, but maintained that more work needed to be done on whether targeting the ECS in humans was a viable treatment option for alcohol use disorder. Few human studies have been conducted to investigate whether medications that target the ECS are effective at treating opioid use disorder, although preliminary data does suggest that dronabinol, a synthetic version of THC, might be helpful for patients with opioid withdrawal. A preclinical study using rats showed that CBD could be useful in preventing relapse induced by environmental cues, while a recent human trial revealed that it could reduce heroin cravings and anxiety in heroin users. The review concluded that more work is needed to investigate whether targeting the ECS could effectively treat substance use disorders, but it did indicate that if research continues to accumulate, the drugs that have been tested could be used in the future "to reduce the public health burden of addiction."[16] Essentially, this means that just because existing treatment options have proven to be more successful than some cannabinoid-based treatments, medications that target the ECS shouldn't be ruled out.

If targeting the body's ECS might have implications for treating addiction to depressants like alcohol and opioids, could the ECS also have implications for addictions to stimulants like cocaine, MDMA, or methamphetamine? A 2013 study by researchers from the University of Montreal, published in *Frontiers in Psychiatry*, asked if cannabinoid-based strategies might have the potential to successfully treat stimulant addiction. In the end, it found that the ECS "reliably modulates relapse to drugs," and that accumulating evidence suggested that the ECS could be a critical target for the development of medications made specifically to treat addiction to stimulants.[17]

A systematic review published in 2015 had more to say about CBD: in looking at nine animal studies and five human studies, it found that CBD might have therapeutic properties in the context of addiction to opioids as well as cocaine and other stimulants, with preliminary data indicating that it could be useful in the treatment of cannabis and tobacco addiction in humans.[18]

While existing evidence is limited and doesn't all support the conclusions of Reiman and many other researchers, we must remember that most studies look at single-compound synthetic medications, and not "cannabis" as we know it. In his latest paper, Canadian researcher Dr. Philippe Lucas argues that increased access to both medical and recreational cannabis has significant positive impacts on public health and safety as a result of what he calls the "substitution effect." With the ongoing opioid crisis in mind, Lucas writes that there are three ways to use cannabis to not only reduce opioid use, but also interrupt the trajectory toward opioid use disorder: (1) in place of opioids in the treatment of chronic pain, (2) as a way to reduce the amount of opioids consumed by a patient who is already using opioids, and (3) as an adjunct therapy alongside methadone or Suboxone, to increase success rates. He writes that the opioid crisis "requires a diversity of novel therapeutic and harm reduction-based interventions, and evidence suggests cannabis may have a role to play in reducing some of these harms."[19]

While Lucas's study looked at therapeutic cannabis use in the context of opiate addiction, the results of it and other bodies of research allow us to draw some conclusions about how cannabis might serve a person caught in the grip of addiction. Cannabis, it seems, has potential in two areas: first, it can provide users with relief from the symptoms of withdrawal, and second, it can serve as an alternative to the addictive substance in question.

Using Cannabis as an Exit Drug

BEFORE WE FLESH out the best ways to consume cannabis as an exit drug, let's consider Lucas's advice on the best times to employ it in the context of opiate addiction. He says that if doctors recommended cannabis *before* suggesting opioids to patients with chronic pain, their patients would be less likely to develop a reliance on or addiction to opioids in the first place. "If physicians and patients have access to a safer, less addictive alternative for pain control like cannabis, introducing it into the course of care as a first line treatment could potentially prevent the opioid overuse cycle from starting," he writes.[20] This places the responsibility of care and of recommending cannabis on the physician, but because many doctors are still hesitant about medical cannabis, it's important that as patients, we ask about our options.

Lucas says that patients already using opioids still have an opportunity to reduce and even cease their use of opioids by using cannabis—but just because you've read that cannabis can help you reduce your opioid consumption, it doesn't mean you should dump your prescriptions down the toilet and go rogue on your doctor.

According to Dr. Perry Solomon, chief medical officer at HelloMD, introducing cannabis is best done under the guidance of a doctor. He warns that it's essential for patients to look to their physicians for oversight, because halting opioid use suddenly can cause more intense withdrawal symptoms than gradually tapering one's use. (Withdrawal symptoms can include tremors, seizures, nausea, insomnia, anxiety, lack of appetite, irritability, and nightmares, and while existing medications aren't quite effective at treating them all at once, cannabis has the ability to address them, though it's incredibly important that a patient reduce their consumption of opioids under the guidance of a medical professional.) While he says there's no magic formula to using cannabis to reduce opioid consumption, he's had patients report that gradually increasing their cannabis use while slowly reducing their opioid consumption not only made withdrawal from opioids more bearable, it also helped relieve the symptoms for which the opioids had originally been prescribed. He says some prefer to use cannabis oil that can be administered under the tongue and is easy to measure in small doses, while others prefer to use capsules.

Every physician who has ever used cannabis to treat addiction will say that recommendations vary from person to person, but generally speaking, people who have never used cannabis before can get by using very low doses of cannabinoids alongside their regular opioid dose to start. Solomon says some patients will find that the cannabis causes the effects of their opioids to become more pronounced, which might make it possible for them to take fewer opioids. Some physicians suggest that tinctures or strains with equal parts THC and CBD could be a good place to start because of their complementary effects, while others prefer to start patients on CBD because of its lack of euphoric effects.

For now, at-home administration in accordance with the guidance of a physician seems to be the most accessible method for replacing opioids with cannabis. While it may feel like cannabis as a medication-assisted treatment for addiction seems far in the future, High Sobriety, a specialized treatment center in Los Angeles, is blazing a new trail by showing evidence of the possibility that the venerable 12-step program might not be the best model when it comes to preventing future relapse. It operates unlike any other treatment center in the world by allowing residents to consume cannabis, eschewing long-standing abstinence models for a program that doesn't force its residents to subscribe to labels of "clean" versus "dirty." When a patient becomes a resident at High Sobriety, they undergo an intake process with a psychiatrist, but unlike a conventional treatment center where patients are prescribed different pharmaceutical agents to help manage their withdrawal, psychiatrists at High Sobriety work with residents to determine how much cannabis is appropriate. It's then administered in the morning, afternoon, and evening, and residents consume it in any way they want, whether that's by smoking, vaporizing, or ingesting it through food or in capsule form. For Reiman, the former clinical research advisor, High Sobriety's success is proof that cannabis should be made available to patients in every treatment center around the world.

THE ENDOCANNABINOID SYSTEM

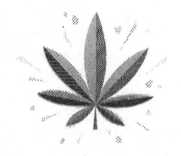

A Discovery for the Ages

FOR CENTURIES, A combination of anecdotal and scientific evidence has pointed to the therapeutic effects of cannabis, with users reportedly experiencing relief from chronic pain; more consistent sleep; a reduction in stress, anxiety, and mood swings; and more—but the data explaining exactly how the various compounds in cannabis actually work in the body has been more challenging to discover.

The scientific breakthrough that would prove to be the first step in explaining what cannabis does in the body was the discovery of the compound tetrahydrocannabinol, or THC, in 1964 by renowned Israeli scientist Dr. Raphael Mechoulam. Shortly after his initial discovery, he and his team were able to identify cannabidiol, or CBD, THC's non-intoxicating counterpart and the second-most abundant compound in cannabis (it's been said that the plant contains as many as four hundred).

"By using a plant that has been around for thousands of years, we discovered a new physiological system of immense importance," said Mechoulam of the event that led to the discovery of the endocannabinoid system.[1]

Unfortunately, it would take decades before scientists were able to make sense of what these compounds did after someone smoked a joint or consumed an edible. In a paper on the discovery of the endocannabinoid system, activist and author Martin A. Lee writes, "Everybody seemed to have an opinion about marijuana, but no one really knew how it worked. . . . No one could explain how cannabis worked as an appetite stimulant, how it dampened nausea, quelled seizures, and relieved pain. . . . No one knew why it lifted one's mood."[2]

It wasn't until 1988 that a study at the St. Louis University School of Medicine found the first cannabinoid receptor—what we now know as CB1—in the brain of a rat. The receptor sites responded to THC and were found in subsequent studies in great numbers throughout the mammalian brain, especially in areas responsible for mental and physiological processes including memory, cognition, motor skills, coordination, and appetite. (Since then, scientists have also found CB1 receptors in humans in the thyroid, liver, reproductive organs, eyes, heart, stomach, pancreas, digestive tract, and muscle.) According to Lee, receptors "function as subtle sensing devices, tiny vibrating scanners perpetually primed to pick up biochemical cues that flow through fluids surrounding each cell."

A few years later, scientists identified what came to be known as the CB2 receptor. This was found throughout the peripheral nervous and immune systems in the gut, spleen, liver, heart, kidneys, bones, lymph cells, endocrine glands, and skin. Where the CB1 receptor, found predominantly in the brain, mediates the psychoactive or euphoric effects of THC, CB2 receptors help regulate the body's immune response.

In 1992, Mechoulam joined forces with William Devane and Dr. Lumír Hanuš from the National Institute of Mental Health (NIMH). They found that the body produced its own compounds that triggered CB1 receptors in the brain and body in the same ways that THC did. They dubbed the naturally occurring compound an endogenous cannabinoid (*endo* meaning internal), and Mechoulam gave it the name anandamide, derived from the Sanskrit word for *bliss*. Three years later, his team discovered a second endogenous cannabinoid, 2-AG, which bound to both CB1 and CB2 receptors. (THC and the endogenous cannabinoids anandamide and 2-AG bind to both varieties of receptors with similar affinity.)

How the Endocannabinoid System Works

. . . .

"THE MAIN INGREDIENT in cannabis closely resembles the way natural endogenous compounds in our body work," says Dr. Ethan Russo, a legendary cannabis researcher and a respected scientist who has been studying the plant for almost thirty years, of this admittedly confusing process by phone from his home in Washington state. "Both THC and anandamide are what are known as partial agonists, meaning they stimulate the CB1 receptors in the brain and throughout the body, throughout the central and peripheral nervous system. What does this mean? If you have too much THC, it's going to be psychoactive, and you might feel high or in the worst manifestations, paranoid or anxious."

While the psychoactive effects of THC get a lot of attention, Russo says it's important not to overlook the manifestation of CB1 receptors elsewhere, especially the way they help stimulate hunger and promote a healthy gut. "A big one it also affects is pain. The endocannabinoid system is one of the main regulators of pain transmission, both in how we perceive it and how we react to it," he says. Russo notes that both THC and CBD are painkillers and have anti-inflammatory properties, but what separates them from opioids and other pain medicines is that they're able to combat pain "in a nonaddictive manner."

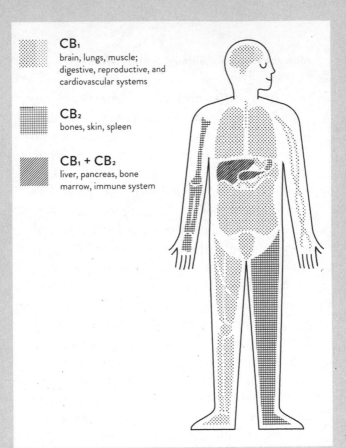

CB₁
brain, lungs, muscle; digestive, reproductive, and cardiovascular systems

CB₂
bones, skin, spleen

CB₁ + CB₂
liver, pancreas, bone marrow, immune system

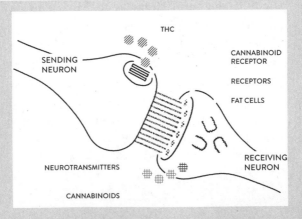

THC

SENDING NEURON

CANNABINOID RECEPTOR

RECEPTORS

FAT CELLS

RECEIVING NEURON

NEUROTRANSMITTERS

CANNABINOIDS

Looking at it from a broader perspective, Russo says the influence of the endocannabinoid system on different aspects of physiological function should not be overlooked. We may have a tendency to focus on its most obvious effects, but it's crucial in far more ways than we tend to give it credit for. Russo notes, "Keep in mind that the endocannabinoid system is everywhere. It's the main homeostatic regulator of our physiology. Let's break that down: *Physiology* is how our various bodily systems work, and *homeostasis* means that we want to have a balance—that the activity is neither too great, nor too little. When we have a balance in the endocannabinoid system, it means that it is working effectively to keep the balance in all these other systems—whether it's emotion, or whether you're about to have a seizure or not, whether it's related to your endocrine system, your digestion, or your hormones—you name it. Everywhere you look in the body, there are mechanisms where the endocannabinoid system helps to keep things regulated and in proper balance."

Achieving that balance can be a challenge, especially when the body isn't producing enough anandamide. While foods high in omega-3 fatty acids can help promote the production of endocannabinoids that will bind to receptors and help return the body to homeostasis, certain enzymes in the body actually work to break down endocannabinoids, adding to the challenge.

The Entourage Effect

....

YOU MIGHT BE wondering where the cannabinoid CBD is in all of this. While THC binds to receptors, CBD interrupts the above-mentioned enzymes from breaking down existing endocannabinoids, increasing the number of naturally occurring compounds like anandamide and 2-AG in the body, and making for a more effective path to homeostasis. This is just one way THC and CBD work together to make each other more effective. As Russo puts it, "CBD helps THC work better." This is the *entourage effect*: the idea that cannabis compounds influence each other's mechanisms.

"Until the last few years, most people ignored the therapeutic value of CBD," Russo says, "but that's not all—there's a whole range of terpenoids, the aromatic compounds in cannabis, which greatly modulate and add to the therapeutic benefits of THC."

The entourage effect is the guiding notion behind the widely held idea that consuming "whole-plant medicine"—that is, a cannabis product derived from a plant in its entirety, and not an isolated compound created in a laboratory—is more beneficial than medication derived from a single compound.

"The best demonstration of this is THC as a standalone synthetic medicine," says Russo. "It's been available in the United States since 1985;

however, it never gained any particular acceptance or market share because THC on its own is a lousy drug!" In his observations, isolated THC causes dysphoria rather than euphoria, and promotes feelings of unhappiness and confusion. He says even people who are experienced with using cannabis tend to find plain THC as Marinol very unpleasant. The benefit of using cannabis products derived from the whole plant is that they contain a variety of other compounds that modulate the effects of THC and "make it more acceptable as a medicine." Foremost among those is CBD.

"When CBD is present, you can give quite a bit more THC without getting the side effect profile that you do when THC is in isolation, and the same is true of terpenoids," Russo says. "They really extend the safety margin of cannabis, specifically the THC content, and contribute to the benefits from a therapeutic standpoint."

HOW TO PREPARE AND USE CANNABIS

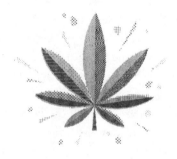

ASK TEN CANNABIS users how they prefer to consume cannabis and you might just get ten different answers. To simplify, I'll break the consumption methods down into four main modalities, and then detail different tools that can be used within those modalities, and what makes them unique. I should note that if you're new to cannabis or you don't consume it regularly, and you're opting to smoke, vaporize, or eat it, START LOW AND GO SLOW. This is the golden rule of cannabis use. If you follow it, you'll reap all the benefits without encountering anxiety or paranoia. This rule is especially applicable if you plan to consume edibles.

Smoking

GRANTED, SMOKING ISN'T going to be your doctor's first choice when you tell them you're interested in trying cannabis, but it's been the preferred method of consumption for thousands of years, and for good reason: smoking cannabis is the quickest way to get the powerful compounds in cannabis to start working right away on what might be ailing you. Cannabinoids enter the body through the lungs and are passed directly into the bloodstream, quickly breaking the blood-brain barrier so that the user feels the effects within minutes. But, as noted above, it's not necessarily the healthiest choice, especially if you want to protect your lungs. While smoking cannabis has nowhere near the same negative effects as smoking cigarettes (likely because people who smoke cannabis don't consume as frequently as those who smoke tobacco), it still does pose some health risks, because cannabis smoke contains tar. Cannabis may not contain the chemical additives used in cigarettes, but the reality is that inhaling smoke can cause irritation of the lungs, skin, and eyes. That being said, studies have shown that cannabis smokers who don't use cigarettes are no more likely than non-cannabis users to develop lung cancer.

Before cannabis can be smoked, it must first be dried and ground. If you're buying your cannabis at a dispensary or through a licensed producer, a good sign of quality is that it comes in "buds" rather than in preground form. (If your cannabis looks like oregano, you've likely been fooled into buying "shake," which is leftover trimmings or bottom-of-the-barrel cannabis better suited to baking than smoking.) Once you've acquired buds, you'll have to invest in a grinder, though in a pinch, a pair of scissors will do—just be warned that other cannabis users in the room might poke fun at your lack of appropriate tools—cannabis users can be snobs when it comes to having the right accessories.

While the joint still remains a popular way to smoke cannabis, hand-rolling a (nice) joint takes lots of practice. Most head shops sell rolling machines at about $5 a pop, but I consider it a fine motor skill worth having. Joints require rolling papers, and, if you prefer not to get cannabis resin on your fingertips and to avoid collecting roaches, a cardboard or glass filter.

If, like a few of my friends, you're either too impatient to roll or you've given up entirely on the sometimes tedious process of perfecting your craft, pipes, bubblers, and bongs can provide an easy way to smoke cannabis. Available in a variety of sizes, materials, styles, prices, and just about any other variable you can think of, these sorts of tools usually consist of a bowl, in which the dried, ground cannabis is placed and lit, and a series of tubes, which the cannabis smoke passes through before it's inhaled.

While there are cannabis users who consider dabbing—a method of consumption that involves inhaling the smoke of a heated (often highly potent)

HOW TO ROLL A JOINT

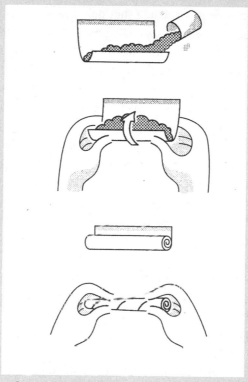

Step 1: Grind cannabis into a fine consistency.

Step 2: Set aside cannabis; roll filter tip into a cylinder.

Step 3: With adhesive side up, sprinkle cannabis onto rolling paper, distributing evenly.

Step 4: Tamp down flower with your fingers. With both hands, use a gentle rolling motion to shape the joint.

Step 5: Slowly tuck the non-adhesive side under the adhesive side. Moisten glue and seal.

Step 6: Insert filter. Twist off the opposite end.

Step 7: Spark, inhale, enjoy.

cannabis concentrate—to be a form of vaporizing, most experts conclude that dabbing is, in fact, a form of smoking, especially when it's done at high temperatures. (As it's been put to me, "anything that leaves char marks on your dab nail is definitely *not* vaporizing.") Dabbing is not for the faint of heart, as it generally involves consuming cannabis concentrates containing upward of 80 percent THC, using high heat and potentially expensive equipment. (That being said, an increasing number of concentrates high in other compounds like CBD and THCA are becoming more popular.) It's definitely not a place for a beginner to start, but, if you're an experienced cannabis user looking for a little extra lift, smoking concentrates like shatter, budder, or rosin can make for next-level euphoria and relaxation that you just can't get from smoking a joint.

Vaporizing

IF YOU'RE NOT interested in combusting the actual plant material, vaporizing provides the same sort of relief, and in the same length of time, without the smoke. When cannabis is vaporized, it is heated to a certain temperature without actually being burned. Vaporizing can be done in a number of ways, either with the same sort of bud used to smoke cannabis, or with a cannabis oil or concentrate that contains higher quantities of THC. Where most cannabis buds can contain anywhere from 5 to 25 percent THC, concentrates can contain more than 80 percent THC, which in turn has a much stronger effect on the body. The ability to use products with higher concentrations is one reason to use a vaporizer, but it's also a favorite for some because it produces almost no odor compared to smoking.

Vaporizers come in many different shapes, sizes, and specialties, from discreet vaporizer pens preloaded with potent oils to handheld machines made to handle both dried buds and concentrates, and of course, the granddaddy of them all, the popular but costly desktop Volcano vaporizer, which allows users to have control of their burn temperature and fill giant balloons with plumes of tasty cannabis vapor. (Don't worry, there are plenty of great, more affordable knock-offs.)

Vaporizers with a temperature control offer users additional benefits, because different cannabis compounds have different boiling points. While THC has a boiling point of roughly 315°F, CBD's boiling point is slightly higher, at 365°F. Some suggest that lower temperatures, say, in the range of 300°F to 330°F, promote a high that is focused, productive, and generally milder. But as your temperatures are increased, the effects of the high become more pronounced. The more you decarboxylate, or activate the THC with heat, the more you activate other compounds in cannabis, including terpenes like myrcene (334°F), limonene (349°F), and linalool (388°F), and cannabinoids like cannabinol, or CBN (365°F), and tetrahydrocannabivarin, or THCV (428°F). A setting between 370°F and 430°F might make for a really nice, relaxing high, but it gets quite close to combustion, and if you're not careful, your cannabis is definitely at risk of burning.

Edibles

EVEN WITH THE option to use a vaporizer, some people just cannot get around the idea of inhaling cannabis. Luckily for them, the key ingredients in cannabis are fat-soluble, making them not only great in food, but also easy to consume in cannabis oils, capsules, and oral sprays. If you live in an area with legal cannabis, finding products to consume orally is easier than ever. What remains difficult for new, and even some experienced, users is pinpointing the right dose.

While the effects of smoking or vaporizing cannabis can be felt quickly, which makes it easy to adjust the dosage on the fly, it takes much longer for cannabis consumed orally to start making its mark. The average cannabis user might expect to wait anywhere from forty-five to ninety minutes to feel the effects of an edible, and people with slower digestive systems might wait several hours before experiencing euphoria. It is for this reason that the rule I stated in all caps at the beginning of this appendix is crucial: if you've spent an hour or so waiting and you're now thinking it might be in your interest to double down on your initial dose, I implore you to resist the urge to consume more cannabis. It's been said that edibles can be the best way to experience cannabis, but also the worst. (Taking too many edibles has made for some hilariously unfortunate personal experiences, and though I never suffered anything worse than some paranoia or an impromptu nap, I've certainly learned the hard way.)

Cannabis consumed orally also elicits a greater "body-stone" effect than smoking or vaporizing, so if you're trying an edible product for the first time, don't plan to do a whole lot. Expect the effects of eating cannabis to be much stronger and to last much longer than smoking or vaporizing.

While some still enjoy taking the homemade route, decarboxylating cannabis in butter or oil and then using it to create infused sauces or bake a batch of "special" brownies, making edibles doesn't necessarily mean you've got to stink up your house, or worse, risk burning perfectly good cannabis while you leave the kitchen to do your laundry. Manufacturers have made it easy, infusing everything—from olive oil to maple syrup and TV dinners to your favorite beverages—with the goodness of cannabis. If you want to consume orally but don't feel the need for an entire infused meal, predosed capsules and tinctures allow you to find the right dose without overdoing it.

Topicals
....................,.

PERSONALLY, I CONSIDER topicals to be a great starting point for individuals with a healthy curiosity about cannabis, because cannabis applied to the skin doesn't cause euphoria. Creams, lotions, roll-ons, lubricants, patches, and my personal favorite—bath bombs—provide a way to experience the anti-inflammatory, analgesic, and relaxing benefits of THC without the high. (Though if you're especially concerned, more and more topical products are being infused with just the nonintoxicating CBD.) These products are formulated to help combat arthritis, aches and pains, inflammation, and skin conditions including acne and psoriasis.

NOTES

• • •

Introduction

1. "Marijuana Arrests by the Numbers," American Civil Liberties Union, updated June 4, 2013, aclu.org/gallery/marijuana-arrests-numbers

2. Alex Luscombe and Akwasi-Owusu-Bempah, "Why Legalization Won't Change Racial Disparities in Cannabis Arrests," VICE News, April 19, 2018, https://news.vice.com/en_ca/article/gymnym/why-legalization-wont-change-racial-disparities-in-cannabis-arrests

3. André Picard, "Canada Needs to Clear the Air—and Wipe Away Records for Marijuana," *Globe and Mail*, January 15, 2018, theglobeandmail.com/cannabis/article-canada-needs-to-clear-the-air-and-wipe-away-criminal-records-for/

Chapter 1

1. "Largest Consumer Sleep Study Ever Released at CES 2017," Sleep score Labs, last modified January 6, 2017, sleepscore.com/news/largest-consumer-sleep-study-ever-released-ces-2017

2. Jean-Philippe Chaput, Suzy L. Wong, and Isabelle Michaud, "Duration and Quality of Sleep among Canadians Aged 18 to 79," *Statistics Canada Health Reports* 28, no. 9 (September 2017): 28-33, www130.statcan.gc.ca/n1/en/pub/82-003-x/2017009/article/54857-eng.pdf?st=uwK_j36y

3. Lawrence Epstein et al., "Improving Sleep: A Guide to a Good Night's Rest," Harvard Medical School (2010): 3-8 (see health.harvard.edu/staying-healthy/improving-sleep-a-guide-to-a-good-nights-rest).

4. Daniel F. Kripke, Robert D. Langer, and Lawrence E. Kline, "Hypnotics' Association with Mortality or Cancer: A Matched Cohort Study," *BMJ Open* 2, no. 1 (2012), bmjopen.bmj.com/content/2/1/e000850

5. William B. O'Shaughnessy, "On the Preparation of the Indian Hemp, or Gunjah (*Cannabis Indica*): Their Effects on the Animal System in Health, and Their Utility in the Treatment of Tetanus and Other Convulsive Diseases," *Provincial Medical Journal and Retrospect of the Medical Sciences* 5, no. 123 (1843): 363–369. Available at ncbi.nlm.nih.gov/pmc/articles/PMC2490264/?page=1

6. Lester Grinspoon and James B. Bakalar, *Marihuana: The Forbidden Medicine* (New Haven: Yale University Press, 1997), 5.

7. "Medical Marijuana Patient Survey Results," HelloMD, January 2016, s3-us-west-2.amazonaws.com/hellomd-news/HelloMD_Medical_Marijuana_Patient_Survey.pdf

8. Zach Walsh et al., "Cannabis for Therapeutic Purposes: Patient Characteristics, Access, and Reasons for Use," *International Journal of Drug Policy* 24, no. 6 (November 2013): 511-516, ijdp.org/article/s0955-3959(13)00135-7/fulltext

9. Nicole P. Bowles, Maya X. Herzig, and Steven A Shea, "Recent Legalization of Cannabis Use: Effects on Sleep, Health, and Workplace Safety," *Nature and Science of Sleep* 9 (October 2017): 249-251, researchgate.net/publication/320513876_Recent_legalization_of_cannabis_use_Effects_on_sleep_health_and_workplace_safety

10. Kenneth Cousens and Alberto DiMascio, "(-)Δ⁹ THC as an Hypnotic," *Psychopharmacologia* 33, no. 4 (December 1973): 355-364, link.springer.com/article/10.1007/BF00437513

11. Bowles et al., "Recent Legalization of Cannabis Use."

12. T. Schierenbeck et al., "Effect of Illicit Recreational Drugs upon Sleep: Cocaine, Ecstasy, and Marijuana," *Sleep Medicine Reviews* 12, no. 5 (October 2008): 381-389, ncbi.nlm.nih.gov/pubmed/18313952

13. Judith Davidson, "Marijuana's Effect on Sleeping Still Unclear," *Globe and Mail*, March 15, 2016, theglobeandmail.com/life/health-and-fitness/health-advisor/marijuanas-effect-on-sleeping-still-unclear/article29247908

14. Elisaldo A. Carlini and Jomar M. Cunha, "Hypnotic and Antiepileptic Effects of Cannabidiol," *Journal of Clinical Pharmacology* 21, no. 8-9 (August-September 1981): 417S-427S, accp1.onlinelibrary.wiley.com/doi/abs/10.1002/j.1552-4604.1981.tb02622.x

15. Anthony Nicholson et al., "Effects of Δ-9 Tetrahydrocannabinol and Cannabidiol on Nocturnal Sleep and Early-Morning Behavior in Young Adults," *Journal of Clinical Psychopharmacology* 24, no. 3 (2004): 305-313, ncbi.nlm.nih.gov/pubmed/15118485

16. Carlini and Cunha, "Hypnotic and Antiepileptic Effects of Cannabidiol."

17. Rakesh Jetley et al., "The Efficacy of Nabilone, a Synthetic Cannabinoid in the Treatment of PTSD-Associated Nightmares: A Preliminary Randomized, Double-Blind, Placebo-Controlled Cross-Over Design Study," *Psychoneuroendocrinology* 51 (January 2015): 585-588, psyneuen-journal.com/article/s0306-4530(14)00413-2/fulltext

18. Michael W. Calik, Miodrag Radulovacki, and David W. Carley, "Intranodose Ganglion Injections of Dronabinol Attenuate Serotonin-Induced Apnea in Sprague-Dawley Rat," *Respiratory Physiology & Neurobiology* 190 (January 2014): 20-24, ncbi.nlm.nih.gov/pmc/articles/PMC3880550

19. Eric Murillo-Rodriguez et al., "Potential Effects of Cannabidiol as a Wake-Promoting Agent," *Current Pharmacology* 12, no. 3 (2014): 269-272, ncbi.nlm.nih.gov/pmc/articles/PMC4023456

Chapter 2

1. "Facts & Statistics," Anxiety and Depression Association of America, adaa.org/about-adaa/press-room/facts-statistics

2. "Stress in America: Coping with Change," American Psychological Association, February 15, 2017, apa.org/news/press/releases/stress/2016/coping-with-change.pdf

3. S. Ruehle et al., "The Endocannabinoid System in Anxiety, Fear Memory and Habituation," *Journal of Psychopharmacology (Oxford, England)* 26, no. 1 (2012): 23-39, ncbi.nlm.nih.gov/pmc/articles/PMC3267552

4. Zach Walsh, Robert Callaway, et al., "Cannabis for Therapeutic Purposes: Patient Characteristics, Access, and Reasons for Use," *International Journal of Drug Policy* 24, no. 6 (November 2013): 511-516, ijdp.org/article/s0955-3959(13)00135-7/fulltext

5. Zach Walsh, Raul Gonzalez, et al., "Medical Cannabis and Mental Health: A Guided Systematic Review," *Clinical Psychology Review* 51 (February 2017): 15-29, sciencedirect.com/science/article/pii/s0272735816300939?via%3Dihub

6. Teniel S. Ramikie et al., "Multiple Mechanistically Distinct Modes of Endocannabinoid Mobilization at Central Amygdala Glutamatergic Synapses," *Neuron* 81, no. 5 (2014): 1111-1125, ncbi.nlm.nih.gov/pmc/articles/PMC3955008

7. José Alexandre S. Crippa, Antonio Waldo Zuardi, and Jaime E. C. Hallak, "Uso terapêutico dos canabinoides em psiquiatria" [Therapeutical use of the cannabinoids in psychiatry] *Revista Brasileira de Psiquiatria* 32, no. 1 (2010): S56-S66, scielo.br/scielo.php?script=sci_arttext&pid=s1516-44462010000500009&lng=en&nrm=iso&tlng=en

8. Isaac G. Karniol et al., "Cannabidiol Interferes with the Effects of Δ^9-Tetrahydrocannabinol in Man," *European Journal of Pharmacology* 28, no. 1 (1974): 172-177, sciencedirect.com/science/article/pii/0014299974901290?via%3Dihub

9. A.W. Zuardi et al., "Action of Cannabidiol on the Anxiety and Other Effects Produced by Δ^9-THC in Normal Subjects," *Psychopharmacology* 76, no. 3 (1982): 245-250, ncbi.nlm.nih.gov/pubmed/6285406

10. Christine A. Rabinak et al., "Cannabinoid Modulation of Prefrontal-Limbic Activation during Fear Extinction Learning and Recall in Humans," *Neurobiology of Learning and Memory* 113 (September 2014): 125-134, ncbi.nlm.nih.gov/pmc/articles/PMC3960373

11. Stephanie M. Gorka et al., "Cannabinoid Modulation of Amygdala Subregion Functional Connectivity to Social Signals of Threat," *International Journal of Neuropsychopharmacology* 18, no. 3 (2015): 1 6, ncbi.nlm.nih.gov/pmc/articles/PMC4360235

12. Edward Wadich, Lisa Y. Adams, and Tony L. Brown, "Neuropsychiatric Effects of Marijuana," *MOJ Addiction Medicine & Therapy* 3 (2017): 61-64, medcraveonline.com/MOJAMT/MOJAMT-03-00034.pdf

13. Esther M. Blessing et al., "Cannabidiol as a Potential Treatment for Anxiety Disorders," *Neurotherapeutics* 12, no. 4 (October 2015): 825-836, ncbi.nlm.nih.gov/pmc/articles/PMC4604171

Chapter 3

1. Canadian Community Health Survey, annual component, "Mood Disorders, by Age Group," Statistics Canada, www150.statcan.gc.ca/t1/tbl1/en/tv.action?pid=1310009618

2. "The Numbers Count: Mental Health Disorders in America," AtHealth, October 23, 2013, athealth.com/topics/the-numbers-count-mental-health-disorders-in-america

3. Matthijs Baas, Carsten K.W. De Dreu, and Bernard A. Nijstad, "A Meta-Analysis of 25 Years of Mood-Creativity Research: Hedonic Tone, Activation, or Regulatory Focus?" *Psychological Bulletin* 134, no. 6 (2008): 779-806, ncbi.nlm.nih.gov/pubmed/18954157

4. Christian Rätsch, *The Encyclopedia of Psychoactive Plants: Ethnopharmacology and Its Applications* (New York: Simon and Schuster, 2005), 138.

5. Jacques-Joseph Moreau, *Hashish and Mental Illness*, trans. Gordon J. Barnett (New York: Raven Press, 1973), 211. Orig. publ. as *Du hachisch et de l'aliénation mentale*, 1845.

6. Chris Bennett, *Cannabis and the Soma Solution* (Walterville: TrineDay LLC, 2010).

7. Zack Walsh et al., "Medical Cannabis and Mental Health: A Guided Systematic Review," *Clinical Psychology Review* 51 (February 2017): 15-29, sciencedirect.com/science/article/pii/s0272735816300939?via%3Dihub

8. Matthijs G. Bossong et al., "The Endocannabinoid System with Emotional Processing: A Pharmacological fMRI Study with Δ9-Tetrahydrocannabinol," *European Neuropsychopharmacology* 23, no. 12 (December 2013): 1687-1697, sciencedirect.com/science/article/pii/s0924977x13001958

9. Mikael A. Kowal et al., "Cannabis and Creativity: Highly Potent Cannabis Impairs Divergent Thinking in Regular Cannabis Users," *Psychopharmacology* 232, no. 6 (2015): 1123-1134, ncbi.nlm.nih.gov/pmc/articles/PMC4336648

10. Emily M. LaFrance and Carrie Cuttler, "Inspired by Mary Jane? Mechanisms Underlying Enhanced Creativity in Cannabis Users," *Consciousness and Cognition* 56 (2017): 68-76, sciencedirect.com/science/article/pii/s1053810017303744?via%3Dihub

Chapter 4

1. Robin Williams, *Live on Broadway*, dir. Marty Callner and Bill Crooks, recorded July 14, 2002, transcript available at script-o-rama.com/movie_scripts/r/robin-williams-live-on-broadway-script.html

2. Nicolas Rodondi et al., "Marijuana Use, Diet, Body Mass Index, and Cardiovascular Risk Factors (from the CARDIA study)," *American Journal of Cardiology* 98, no. 4 (2006): 478-484, ajconline.org/article/s0002-9149(06)00817-4/fulltext

3. Denise C. Vidot et al., "Metabolic Syndrome among Marijuana Users in the United States: An Analysis of National Health and Nutrition Examination Survey Data," *American Journal of Medicine* 129, no. 2 (February 2016): 173-189, ncbi.nlm.nih.gov/pmc/articles/PMC4718895

4. Vidot et al., "Metabolic Syndrome among Marijuana Users in the United States."

5. Lexie Zhiyan Jin et al., "Association between Use of Cannabis in Adolescence and Weight Change into Midlife," *PLOS One* 12, no. 1 (2017): e0168897, journals.plos.org/plosone/article?id=10.1371/journal.pone.0168897

6. Hilal Ahmad Parray and Jong Won Yun, "Cannabidiol Promotes Browning in 3T3-L1 Adipocytes," *Molecular and Cellular Biochemistry* 416, no. 1-2 (May 2016): 131-139, link.springer.com/article/10.1007%2Fs11010-016-2702-5

7. Ethan B. Russo, "Taming THC: Potential Cannabis Synergy and Phytocannabinoid-Terpenoid Entourage Effects," *British Journal of Pharmacology* 163, no. 7 (2011): 1344-1364, ncbi.nlm.nih.gov/pmc/articles/PMC3165946

8. Gernot Riedel et al., "Synthetic and Plant-Derived Cannabinoid Receptor Antagonists Show Hypophagic Properties in Fasted and Non-Fasted Mice," *British Journal of Pharmacology* 156, no. 7 (April 2009): 1154-1156, ncbi.nlm.nih.gov/pmc/articles/PMC2697695

9. Dominik H. Pesta et al., "The Effects of Caffeine, Nicotine, Ethanol, and Tetrahydrocannabinol on Exercise Performance," *Nutrition & Metabolism* 10, no. 71 (2013): 1-15, ncbi.nlm.nih.gov/pmc/articles/PMC3878772

10 R.D. Steadward and M. Singh, "The Effects of Smoking Marihuana on Physical Performance," *Medicine & Science in Sports & Exercise* 7, no. 4 (1975): 309-311, ncbi.nlm.nih.gov/pubmed/1235156

11. Edward V. Avakian et al., "Effect of Marihuana on Cardiorespiratory Responses to Submaximal Exercise," *Clinical Pharmacology & Therapeutics* 26, no. 6 (1979): 777-781, ncbi.nlm.nih.gov/pubmed/498720

12. Pesta et al., "The Effects of Caffeine."

13. Maria B. Brisola-Santos et al., "Prevalence and Correlates of Cannabis Use among Athletes—A Systematic Review," *American Journal on Addictions* 25, no. 7 (October 2016): 518-528, ncbi.nlm.nih.gov/pubmed/27629700

14. Brisola-Santos et al., "Prevalence and Correlates of Cannabis Use among Athletes."

Chapter 5

1. Christy Brissette, "Milk, Bread, Hemp Oil? A Dietitian's Guide to the Cannabis Items in Your Grocery Store," *Washington Post*, April 20, 2018, washingtonpost.com/lifestyle/wellness/milk-bread-hemp-oil-a-dietitians-guide-to-the-cannabis-items-in-your-grocery-store/2018/04/19/c7fb1dd8-43d7-11e8-bba2-0976a82b05a2_story.html?utm_term=.2a07b11cee25

2. Jack Herer, *The Emperor Wears No Clothes: The Authoritative Historical Record of Cannabis and the Conspiracy against Marijuana* (Van Nuys: Ah Ha Publishing, 1985), 71.

3. Ken Albala, *Cooking in Europe, 1250-1650* (Westport: Greenwood, 2006), 73.

4. Albala, *Cooking in Europe*.

5. Karl Vick, "Form of Medical Marijuana Won't Get You High, but It's Creating a Buzz," *Washington Post*, June 1, 2010, washingtonpost.com/wp-dyn/content/article/2010/05/31/AR2010053103231.html

6. Marisa Crane, "What Does a Marijuana Overdose Look Like?" *Project Know: Understanding Addiction*, projectknow.com/research/marijuana-overdose

Chapter 6

1. Ethan B. Russo, Melanie Dreher, and Mary Lynn Mathre, *Women and Cannabis: Medicine, Science, and Sociology* (New York: The Haworth Herbal Press, 2002), 75.

2. Michael R. Aldrich, "Tantric Cannabis Use in India," *Journal of Psychedelic Drugs* 9, no. 3 (1977): 227-233, researchgate.net/publication/233211369_Tantric_Cannabis_Use_in_India

3. Robert C. Clarke and Mark D. Merlin, *Cannabis: Evolution and Ethnobotany* (Berkeley: University of California Press, 2013), 260.

4. William B. O'Shaughnessy, quoted by E.W. Berridge, "Cannabis Indica," *The Homeopathic World: A Popular Journal of Medical, Social, and Sanitary Science* 14 (January 1, 1879): 119-124.

5. Sula Benet, "Early Diffusion and Folk Uses of Hemp," in *Cannabis and Culture*, ed. Vera Rubin (The Hague: Mouton, 1975), 39-49.

6. Maud Kamatenesi-Mugisha and Hannington Oryem-Origa, "Traditional Herbal Remedies Used in the Management of Sexual Impotence and Erectile Dysfunction in Western Uganda," *African Health Sciences* 5, no. 1 (2005): 40-49, ncbi.nlm.nih.gov/pmc/articles/PMC1831906

7. Wayne C. Koff, "Marijuana and Sexual Activity," *Journal of Sex Research* 10, no. 3 (1974): 194-204, researchgate.net/publication/18697057_Marijuana_and_sexual_activity

8. Ronald A. Weller and James A. Halikas, "Marijuana Use and Sexual

Behavior," *Journal of Sex Research* 20, no. 2 (May 1984): 186-193, jstor.org/stable/3812350?seq=1#page_scan_tab_contents

9. Tina Djernis Gundersen et al., "Association between Use of Marijuana and Male Reproductive Hormones and Semen Quality: A Study among 1,215 Healthy Young Men," *American Journal of Epidemiology* 182, no. 6 (September 2015): 473-381, academic.oup.com/aje/article/182/6/473/82600

10. Richard Balon, "Cannabis and Sexuality," *Current Sexual Health Reports* 9, no. 3 (September 2017): 99-103, deepdyve.com/lp/springer-journals/cannabis-and-sexuality-XjlD20ln5j

11. Andrew J. Sun and Michael L. Eisenberg, "Association between Marijuana Use and Sexual Frequency in the United States: A Population-Based Study," *Journal of Sexual Medicine* 14, no. 11 (2017): 1342-1347, ncbi.nlm.nih.gov/pubmed/29110804

Chapter 7

1. Committee on Advancing Pain Research, Care, and Education, *Relieving Pain in America: A Blueprint for Transforming Prevention, Care, and Research* (Washington: The National Academies Press, 2011), 55-112, nap.edu/read/13172/chapter/1

2. "Global Pain Management Market to Reach US$60 Billion by 2015, according to a New Report by Global Industry Analysts, Inc.," PR Web, last modified January 10, 2011, prweb.com/releases/2011/1/prweb8052240.htm

3. "NIH Analysis Shows Americans Are in Pain," National Center for Complementary and Integrative Health, last modified August 11, 2015, nccih.nih.gov/news/press/08112015

4. "Chronic Pain: Symptoms, Diagnosis, & Treatment," National Institutes of Health Medline Plus, last modified spring 2011, medlineplus.gov/magazine/issues/spring11/articles/spring11pg5-6.html

5. "AAPM: Facts and Figures on Pain," American Academy of Pain Medicine, painmed.org/files/facts-and-figures-on-pain.pdf

6. Uwe Blesching, *The Cannabis Health Index: Combining the Science of Medical Marijuana with Mindfulness Techniques to Heal 100 Chronic Symptoms and Diseases* (Berkeley: North Atlantic Books, 2015), 405.

7. Ethan B. Russo and Andrea G. Hohmann, "Role of Cannabinoids in Pain Management," in *Comprehensive Treatment of Chronic Pain by Medical, Interventional, and Integrative Approaches*, eds. Timothy R. Deer et al. (New York: Springer, 2013), 181-98.

8. Ernest L. Abel, *Marijuana: The First Twelve Thousand Years* (New York: Plenum Press, 1980), 12.

9. Cited by Lumír O. Hanuš, "Discovery and Isolation of Anandamide and Other Endocannabinoids," *Chemistry & Biodiversity* 4, no. 8 (2007): 1828-1841, onlinelibrary.wiley.com/doi/abs/10.1002/cbdv.200790154

10. Cited by R.D. Hosking and J.P. Zajicek, "Therapeutic Potential of Cannabis in Pain Medicine," *British Journal of Anaesthesia* 101, no. 1 (2008): 59-68, bjanaesthesia.org/article/s0007-0912(17)34269-1/fulltext

11. Gabriel G. Nahas and Albert Greenwood, "The First Report of the National Commission on Marihuana (1972): Signal of Misunderstanding or Exercise in Ambiguity," *Bulletin of the New York Academy of Medicine* 50, no. 1 (1974): 55-75, ncbi.nlm.nih.gov/pmc/articles/PMC1749335

12. Kevin P. Hill et al., "Cannabis and Pain: A Clinical Review," *Cannabis and Cannabinoid Research* 2, no. 1 (2017): 96-104, ncbi.nlm.nih.gov/pmc/articles/PMC5549367

13. Hill et al., "Cannabis and Pain."

14. Russo and Hohmann, "Role of Cannabinoids in Pain Management."

15. Mark A. Ware et al., "Cannabis for the Management of Pain: Assessment of Safety Study (COMPASS)," *Journal of Pain* 16, no. 12 (2015): 1233-1242, jpain.org/article/s1526-5900(15)00837-8/fulltext

Chapter 8

1. "Cancer Facts & Figures 2018," American Cancer Society, last modified 2018, cancer.org/content/dam/cancer-org/research/cancer-facts-and-statistics/annual-cancer-facts-and-figures/2018/cancer-facts-and-figures-2018.pdf

2. Rebecca L. Siegel, Kimberly D. Miller, and Ahmedin Jemal, "Cancer Statistics, 2018," *CA: A Cancer Journal for Clinicians* 68, no. 1 (2018): 7-30, onlinelibrary.wiley.com/doi/full/10.3322/caac.21442

3. "Canadian Cancer Statistics 2017," Canadian Cancer Society, last modified June 2017, cancer.ca/~/media/cancer.ca/cw/publications/Canadian%20cancer%20statistics/Canadian-Cancer-Statistics-2017-EN.pdf

4. Akulapalli Sudhakar, "History of Cancer, Ancient and Modern Treatment Methods," *Journal of Cancer Science & Therapy* 1, no. 2 (2009): 1-4, ncbi.nlm.nih.gov/pmc/articles/PMC2927383

5. Ethan B. Russo, "History of Cannabis and Its Preparations in Saga, Science, and Sobriquet," *Chemistry & Biodiversity* 4, no. 8 (2007): 1614-1648, pdfs.semanticscholar.org/d7b0/d0fbeb02be9cef8e0bbc4df3d228762dc12d.pdf?_ga=2.98482395.531888725.1529872555-1926093065.1529872555

6. Albert E. Munson et al., "Antineoplastic Activity of Cannabinoids," *Journal of the National Cancer Institute* 55, no. 3 (1975): 597-602, ncbi.nlm.nih.gov/pubmed/1159836

7. Kambiz Akhavan, "Marinol vs. Marijuana: Politics, Science, and Popular Culture," The American Alliance for Medical Cannabis, 1997, letfreedomgrow.com/articles/marinolvsmarijuana.htm

8. "Drug Schedules," United States Drug Enforcement Administration, dea.gov/druginfo/ds.shtml

9. Bakht Nasir et al., "Cannabis: A Prehistoric Remedy for the Deficits of Existing and Emerging Anticancer Therapies," *Journal of Exploratory Research in Pharmacology* 2, no. 3 (2017): 93-104, xiahepublishing. com/2572-5505/ArticleFullText.aspx?sid=2&id=10.14218%2fJERP. 2017.00012

10. Sofía Torres et al., "A Combined Preclinical Therapy of Cannabinoids and Temozolomide against Glioma," *Molecular Cancer Therapeutics* 10, no. 1 (2011): 90-103, mct.aacrjournals.org/content/10/1/90.long

11. D.I. Abrams, "Integrating Cannabis into Clinical Cancer Care," *Current Oncology* 23, no. S2 (2016): S8-S14, ncbi.nlm.nih.gov/ pubmed/27022315

12. Carolyn Crist, "The Doctor Will See You Now—but Not for Long," Reuters, November 28, 2017, reuters.com/article/us-doctor-checkup- duration/the-doctor-will-see-you-now-but-often-not-for-long- idUSKBN1DS2Z2

Chapter 9

1. "Dementia Statistics," Alzheimer's Disease International, last modified May 16, 2017, alz.co.uk/research/statistics

2. Jonathon Green, *Cannabis* (London: Pavilion, 2002), 178.

3. Nicholas Culpeper, *The English Physician* (Tuscaloosa: University of Alabama Press, 2007), 91. Orig. publ. 1708.

4. Megan Weier and Wayne Hall, "The Use of Cannabinoids in Treating Dementia," *Current Neurology and Neuroscience Reports* 17, no. 8 (2017), link.springer.com/article/10.1007%2Fs11910-017-0766-6

5. Chuanhai Cao et al., "The Potential Therapeutic Effects of THC on Alzheimer's Disease," *Journal of Alzheimer's Disease* 42, no. 3 (2014): 974-984, content.iospress.com/articles/journal-of-alzheimers- disease/jad140093

6. Lisa M. Eubanks et al., "A Molecular Link between the Active Com- ponent of Marijuana and Alzheimer's Disease Pathology," *Molecular Pharmaceutics* 3, no. 6 (2006): 773-777, ncbi.nlm.nih.gov/pmc/ articles/PMC2562334

7. Antonio Currais et al., "Amyloid Proteotoxicity Initiates an Inflamma- tory Response Blocked by Cannabinoids," *Aging and Mechanisms of Disease* 2 (2016): 1-8, 16012, nature.com/articles/npjamd201612

8. Andras Bilkei-Gorzo et al., "A Chronic Low Dose of Δ9-Tetrahydro- cannabinol (THC) Restores Cognitive Function in Old Mice," *Nature Medicine* 23, no. 6 (June 2017): 782-787, nature.com/articles/nm.4311

9. Brian Kaskie et al., "The Increasing Use of Cannabis among Older Americans: A Public Health Crisis or Viable Policy Alternative?" *The Gerontologist* 57, no. 6 (November 10, 2017): 1166-1172, academic.oup. com/gerontologist/article-lookup/doi/10.1093/geront/gnw166

Chapter 10

1. "The Science of Drug Abuse and Addiction: The Basics," [Media Guide], National Institute on Drug Abuse, last modified October 1, 2016, drugabuse.gov/publications/media-guide/science-drug-abuse-addiction-basics

2. "Opioid Overdose: Understanding the Epidemic," Centers for Disease Control and Prevention, last modified August 30, 2017, cdc.gov/drugoverdose/epidemic

3. Sheila Kaplan, "C.D.C. Reports a Record Jump in Drug Overdose Deaths Last Year," *The New York Times*, November 3, 2017, nytimes.com/2017/11/03/health/deaths-drug-overdose-cdc.html

4. Camille Bains, "B.C. Officials Consider Options after 88 per cent Increase in Overdose Deaths," *Maclean's*, August 5, 2017, macleans.ca/news/canada/b-c-officials-consider-options-after-88-per-cent-increase in-overdose-deaths/

5. "Marijuana: Is Marijuana Addictive?" National Institute on Drug Abuse, last modified May 2018, drugabuse.gov/publications/research-reports/marijuana/marijuana-addictive

6. See Introduction.

7. "Drugs of Abuse: A DEA Resource Guide—2017 Edition," Drug Enforcement Administration, U.S. Department of Justice, dea.gov/pr/multimedia-library/publications/drug_of_abuse.pdf

8. Cited in Tod H. Mikuriya, "Cannabis as a Substitute for Alcohol: A Harm-Reduction Approach," *Journal of Cannabis Therapeutics* 4, no. 1 (2004): 79-93, cannabis-med.org/iacm/data/pdf/2004-01-3.pdf

9. Tod H. Mikuriya, ed., *Marijuana: Medical Papers, 1839-1972* (Oakland: Medi-Comp Press, 1973), xiii-xxvii.

10. Amanda Reiman, "Cannabis as a Substitute for Alcohol and Other Drugs," *Harm Reduction Journal* 6, no. 35 (2009), harmreductionjournal.biomedcentral.com/articles/10.1186/1477-7517-6-35

11. Philippe Lucas et al., "Cannabis as a Substitute for Alcohol and Other Drugs: A Dispensary-Based Survey of Substitution Effect in Canadian Medical Cannabis Patients," *Addiction Research & Theory* 21, no. 5 (2013): 435-442, tandfonline.com/doi/abs/10.3109/16066359.2012.733465

12. Amanda Reiman, Mark Welty, and Perry Solomon, "Cannabis as a Substitute for Opioid-Based Pain Medication: Patient Self-Report," *Cannabis and Cannabinoid Research* 2, no. 1 (2017): 160-166, liebertpub.com/doi/full/10.1089/can.2017.0012

13. Yuyan Shi, "Medical Marijuana Policies and Hospitalizations Related to Marijuana and Opioid Pain Reliever," *Drug and Alcohol Dependence* 173 (April 2017): 144-150, ncbi.nlm.nih.gov/pubmed/28259087

14. Melvin D. Livingston et al., "Recreational Cannabis Legalization and Opioid-Related Deaths in Colorado, 2000–2015," *American Journal of Public Health* 107, no. 11 (November 2017): 1827–1829, ncbi.nlm.nih.gov/pubmed/29019782

15. Matthew E. Sloan et al., "The Endocannabinoid System as a Target for Addiction Treatment: Trials and Tribulations," *Neuropharmacology* 124 (September 2017): 73–83, sciencedirect.com/science/article/pii/S0028390817302563?via%3Dihub

16. Sloan et al., "The Endocannabinoid System."

17. Stéphanie Olière et al., "Modulation of the Endocannabinoid System: Vulnerability Factor and New Treatment Target for Stimulant Addiction," *Frontiers in Psychiatry* 4 (September 2013): 1–21, ncbi.nlm.nih.gov/pmc/articles/PMC3780360

18. Mélissa Prud'homme, Romulus Cata, and Didier Jutras-Aswad, "Cannabidiol as an Intervention for Addictive Behaviors: A Systematic Review of the Evidence," *Substance Abuse* 9 (May 2015): 33–38, ncbi.nlm.nih.gov/pmc/articles/PMC4444130

19. Philippe Lucas, "Rationale for Cannabis-Based Interventions in the Opioid Overdose Crisis," *Harm Reduction Journal* 14 (2017): 1–6, article 58, harmreductionjournal.biomedcentral.com/articles/10.1186/s12954-017-0183-9

20. Lucas, "Rationale for Cannabis-Based Interventions."

Appendix 1

1. Martin A. Lee, "The Discovery of the Endocannabinoid System," Beyond THC, last modified 2012, beyondthc.com/wp-content/uploads/2012/07/eCBSystemLee.pdf

2. Lee, "The Discovery of the Endocannabinoid System."

ACKNOWLEDGMENTS

• • •

Without the expertise and lived experience provided to me by the voices in this book, and the care and consideration of a core group of people, there is no way I could have finished it.

To experts Dr. Perry Solomon, Dr. Jeremy Spiegel, Dr. Carrie Cuttler, Dr. Denise Vidot, Robin Griggs Lawrence, Ashley Manta, Dr. Mark Ware, Dr. Bryn Hyndman, Mara Gordon, Dr. Brian Kaskie, Dr. Amanda Reiman, and Dr. Ethan Russo, whose generosity with both their time and their knowledge utterly exceeded my expectations: thank you for your enthusiasm for my questions and your eagerness to speak truthfully to what cannabis can do. I am both awed and inspired by your work and so happy to include your words in this book.

A special thank-you to Dr. Zach Walsh, who has always been available when I've had questions for a story about cannabis and mental health: not only did your words make sense of research on a topic that can sometimes present different conclusions, they also helped me understand my own post-traumatic stress disorder when I wasn't able to see what was really going on. The impact of that discussion was profound, to say the least.

Endless gratitude to Guilherme Falcão, Piper Courtenay, Jon Bent, Ross Rebagliati, Mary Jean "Watermelon" Dunsdon, Lisa "Mamakind" Kirkman, Galen Pallas, Alan Park, Selena Wong, and Siobhan McCarthy. Your stories help make the material in this book come to life. Thank you for being uninhibited, for trusting me with your experiences, and for the work that you do to help destigmatize a plant with an undeserved reputation.

To Dr. Rav Ivker: I read your book, *Cannabis for Chronic Pain*, during my initial research and was so overjoyed to learn you were writing a foreword for me. Thank you for your kind words, your passionate work, and your focus on patients.

Many, many thanks to Jen Croll, whose carefully crafted idea spoke to my passion for medical cannabis so well. You made the first-time author experience far more pleasant than my anxious mind allowed and even on a tight schedule you found ways for me to take extra time when my health didn't seem to care about deadlines.

A special thank-you to Eva van Emden and Lesley Cameron for your thoughtful and thorough edits, to Dawn Loewen for proofreading, and to Jen Gauthier, Alice Fleerackers, Josh Oliviera, and the rest of the Greystone team for your marketing

THE LITTLE BOOK OF CANNABIS

chops. I'm so grateful for the work of the artists and designers who have contributed: thank you to Brian Tong for your illustrations and cover design, and to Nayeli Jimenez for your work inside the book. To publisher Rob Sanders, thank you for believing in this idea in its earliest stages.

Thank you to my former editors and colleagues at the *Straight*, who had faith in my writing ability and gave me the perfect balance of guidance and freedom; to my friends and colleagues in the Vancouver cannabis community for your endless support; and to local readers who have engaged with my work.

Many thanks to the strong women in my life who have always led by example—particularly to Andrea Isaak, for your kick-ass-and-take-names, take-no-shit attitude (and for telling me long ago at that piano bench that one day I'd write a book). A special thank-you to my younger-but-wiser brother, Daniel, and of course, to my mom and dad: while I will continue to pray for the day we can stand side by side at a backyard barbecue and share a joint, I am grateful that you have accepted me for the loud, cussing, pink-haired, pot-smoking individual that I am. Your lessons of hard work and constant love and support surely laid the foundation for the woman I've become.

To my best friend Eric Ng: "Thank you" doesn't feel like enough. Thank you for giving me all the patience, consideration, and kindness I needed to see this task through to completion, and for bringing rationality and peace to my mind when I thought my mind itself had been lost. Most of all, thank you for believing in me when I felt like I couldn't believe in myself.

Finally, to the readers who've made it to the end: Thank you for opening your mind to the possibility that cannabis can in fact be a source of *positive* in your life. I'm grateful for your willingness to shift your perspective, and my hope is that together, we can share the truth about a plant whose undeserved reputation needs to finally be shed.